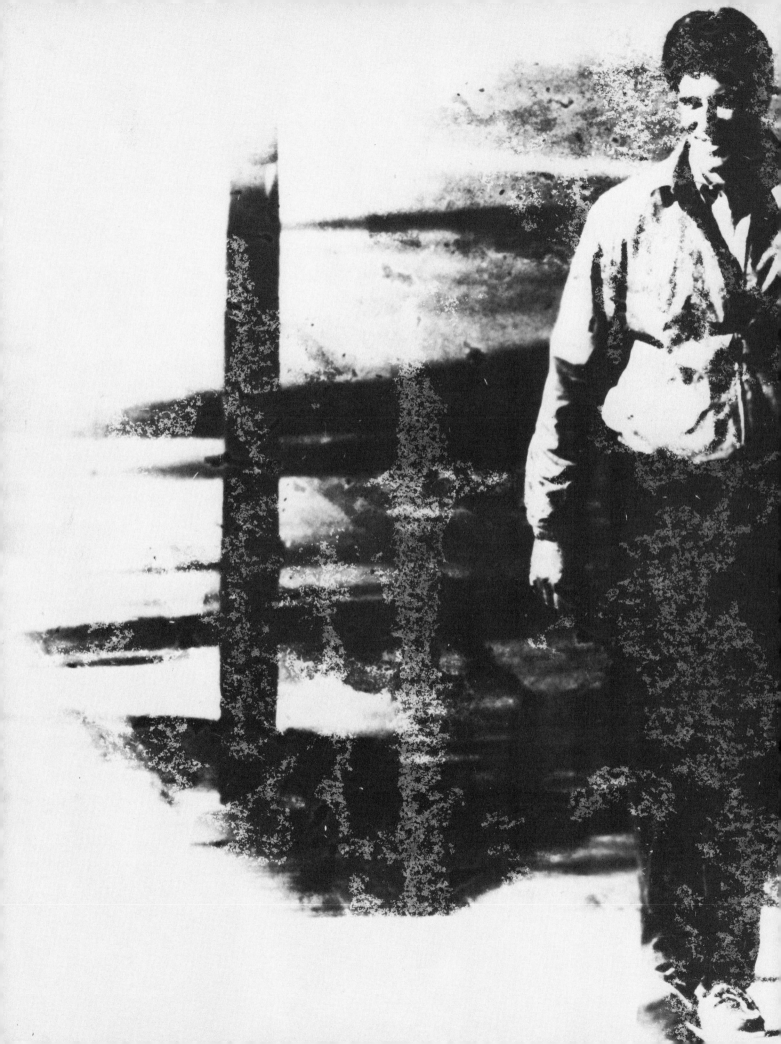

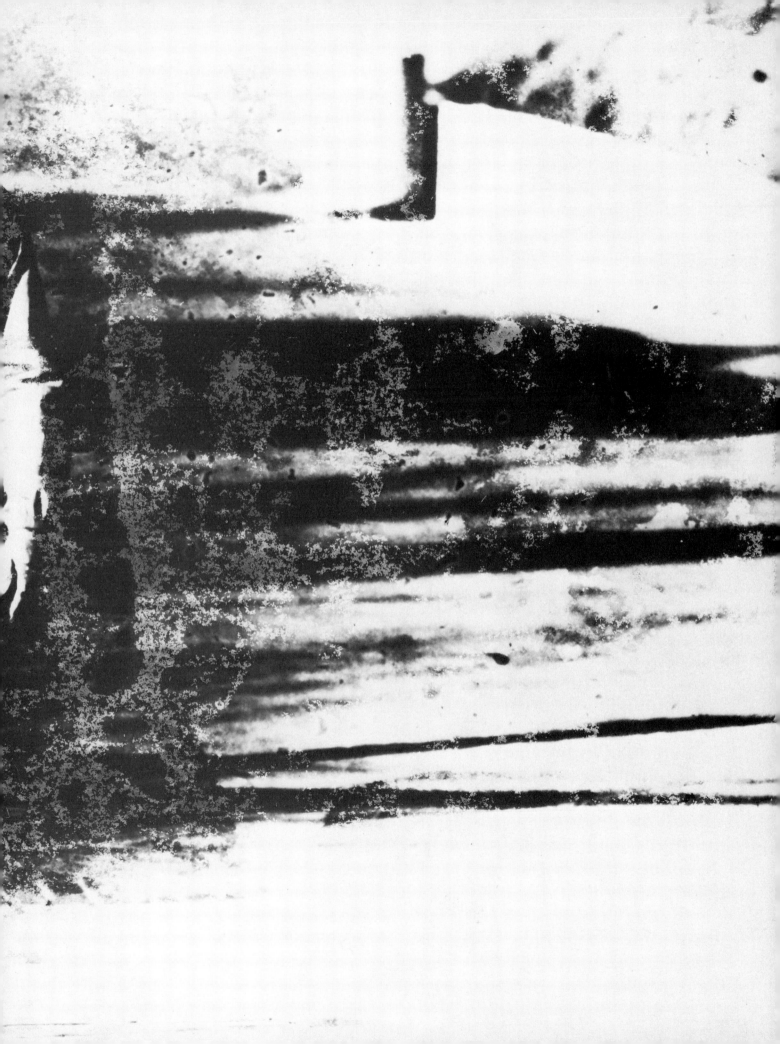

JIM PALMER'S WAY TO FITNESS

JIM PALMER'S WAY TO FITNESS

by Jim Palmer

with Jack Clary

Photography by Jon Naso, Sports Action Photography, Princeton, New Jersey

Exercise Programs by Nancy L. Siegel, RPT

1817

Harper & Row, Publishers, New York
Cambridge, Philadelphia, San Francisco
London, Mexico, São Paulo, Singapore, Sydney

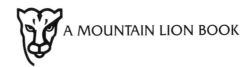
A MOUNTAIN LION BOOK

FIRST EDITION

Designers: Dilip Kane, Richard Vitti, and Bill Pasiliavich

Library of Congress Cataloging in Publication Data

Palmer, Jim, 1945-
   Jim Palmer's way to fitness.

   Includes index.
   1. Physical fitness.   I. Clary, Jack.   II. Title.
III. Title: Way to fitness.
GV481.P314 1985   613.7   84-48187
ISBN 0-06-015407-1

85 86 87 88 89 10 9 8 7 6 5 4 3 2 1

CONTENTS

1. The Jim Palmer Way to Fitness: **1**
   Shape Up Your Body, Change Your Life

2. Palmerfit Program: **7**
   Loosening Up, Working Out, Cooling Down

3. Playing Sports to Stay Fit...   **37**
   But Let's Not Get Hurt

4. Body Balance and Posture: **69**
   Stand Straight, Walk Tall

5. Nutritional Edge: **79**
   Balancing Good Times and Good Food

6. The Personal Touch: **93**
   Hair and Skin Care

7. Fashion Fit: **107**
   Smart Dressing for All Occasions

8. Bottom of the Ninth; Bases Loaded,   **121**
   Two Outs and Full Count...
   or How to Handle Stress

9. Epilogue: Jim Palmer—The Private Person,   **133**
   The Public Performer

   Appendix I   Common Muscle Discomforts   **149**

   Appendix II   Calorie Chart   **151**

   Index   **159**

   Acknowledgements   **167**

JIM PALMER'S WAY TO FITNESS

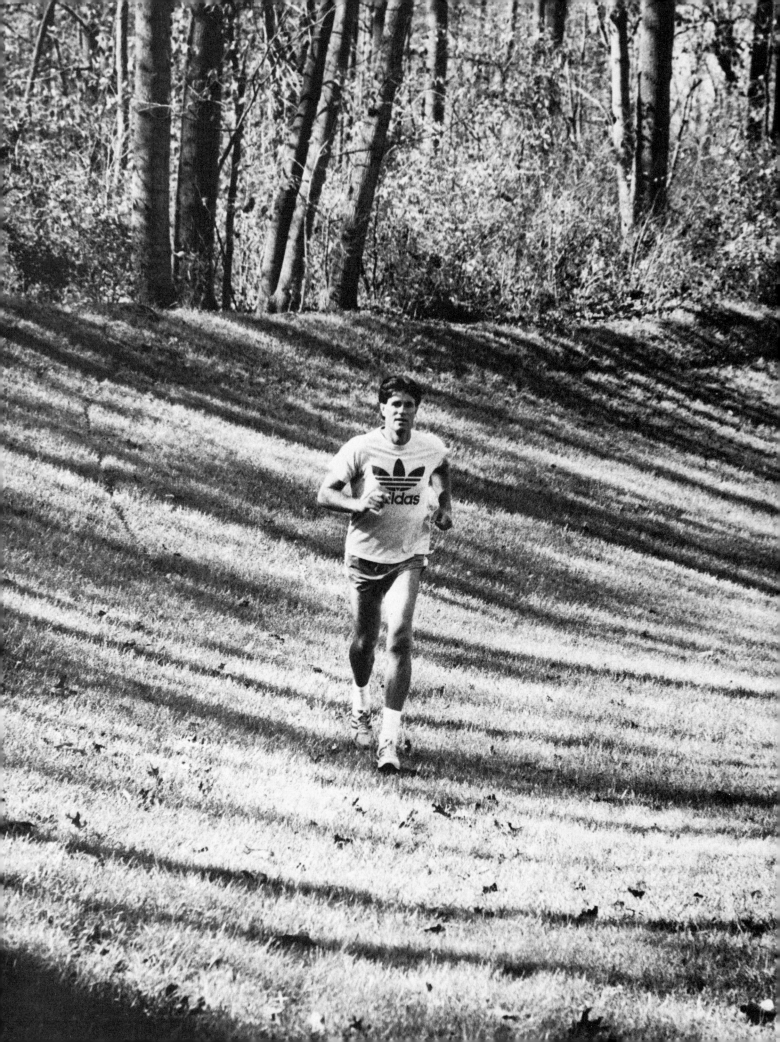

THE JIM PALMER WAY TO FITNESS: SHAPE UP YOUR BODY, CHANGE YOUR LIFE

1967 was one of the worst years in my life. My major-league pitching career, which had gotten off to such a great start when I had helped the Baltimore Orioles win the 1966 World Championship, was at a serious crossroads. I kept having pain and stiffness in my pitching arm; nothing seemed to help. I had missed a season, and I really wasn't sure I'd ever be able to pitch again.

It was decided that I would undergo a physical-conditioning program at a Baltimore hospital in an attempt to cure the problem. I had always taken pretty good care of myself, or at least I thought I had, but this program was unlike anything I'd ever done before.

Now, a funny thing happened on the way to repairing my arm—it didn't work as I had hoped, at least not then. But something just as good came from it: a realization of the benefits of a consistent physical-fitness regimen. When my arm problem later disappeared, I resumed my pitching career with very satisfactory results.

As a professional baseball player, particularly as a pitcher, it was absolutely necessary that I do something to stay more than just fit. Baseball may seem like a physically lax game for those who watch it, but for those who play it, it involves a great deal of physical stress. That is why I determined to work year-round to have my body in the best possible shape instead of waiting until spring training to do the job—which was the norm back when I had my arm problem as a young pitcher.

The results soon became apparent away from the field as well. I needed a fitness program to feel good ... so I stayed with it to feel good.

I am nearing forty—half of my life has been spent pitching in the major leagues. I've often asked myself: "How did I last for twenty years, for more than four thousand innings?"

Not without working at it (and keeping that fast ball in a good location). I did work at it. In fact, last fall during a visit with my good friend and former teammate Davey Leonhard, he said to me, ''You could still pitch. You never abused yourself and you live an active, physically fit life.''

Well, I have few illusions about ever pitching again, but I can't argue with Davey about the way I maintain my fitness. Though my baseball career is over, this has become so ingrained that I have no intention of slackening off and ''relaxing a little.'' I simply cannot work well as national spokesman for Jockey and in broadcasting, with all of the travel, preparation and in-person demands, unless I am feeling fit.

I believe that if this is my experience, then it is true for you, too. Enough people have asked about staying fit and the impact it has on my life to convince me that this is a nationwide concern.

There are a lot of exercise books. What's different about my program? The workouts that

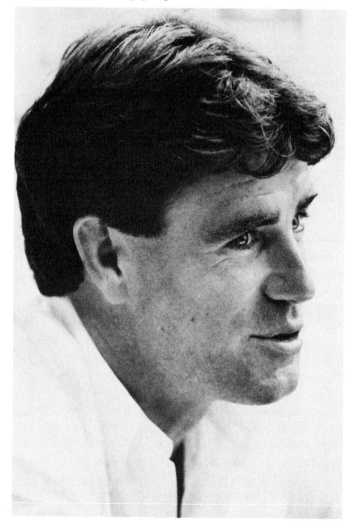

follow represent a *balanced system*. They provide muscular strength and endurance, and cardiovascular fitness. My program is not tied to any one activity, such as running or jogging, but offers you the option of freely substituting other activities, such as swimming or cycling, that provide similar benefits.

This program is not expensive to begin or maintain. Little or no equipment is necessary. You can begin in your own home on the living-room floor. I have set forth an injury-free routine: warmup, exercise and cooldown. This adheres to the body's natural cycle of physical activity, which is universally prescribed by expert physiologists but is often overlooked or not emphasized in other exercise programs. And although the sections of this book on hair and skin care and how to dress are directed to the specific needs of men, the exercise programs and nutrition guidelines can be followed by both men and women.

I try to live fit and to think fit, but that doesn't mean I won't have an occasional glass of wine.

Now, I am not a zealot who believes that all there is to life is exercising morning, noon and night, and that you somehow are cheating yourself if you enjoy some treats. I try to live fit and to think fit, but that doesn't mean I won't have an occasional glass of wine before dinner or at a party, or that I'll never indulge myself in my favorite chocolate-chip cookies.

Yet, if you have not been attentive to the type of living routine which I will be suggesting throughout this book, then I am asking you to adopt what will be, in great measure, a new lifestyle. It will not be sackcloth and ashes, by any means, but it may be different—and to some of you, *very, very* different.

You must make a conscious effort if you are to follow the three commandments which will be your guide throughout this program:

- Think fit!
- Do something about it!
- And keep doing something about it!

If you have any doubts about these aims, take a good look at yourself in a full-length mirror. Are you happy with what you see? Or away from that mirror, are you happy with how you physically feel? Think over those two questions because only you can answer them honestly.

Now I'll ask you another: What can you hope to get out of this book, that might provide the solutions you are seeking?

You will find a way to exercise to look better, and a way to exercise to feel better.

And there will be even more.

If you follow the exercise program that follows, you not only will feel better but your circulation will improve ... your heart rate will be lower ... you will sleep better ... you will work better ... you will be more productive ... you may well add years to your life and certainly its quality will improve. Your sense of personal well-being will increase because you will feel good about having forced yourself to do something you never did before, and forced yourself to stay with it during the times when you wanted to quit—and there may be plenty of those.

I believe those are sufficiently good reasons to make the necessary commitments and put up with the temporary inconveniences. Once you take this entire fitness program to heart and make it a part of your daily routine, those rough spots will completely disappear.

I'm sure there are some of you who think that because you play tennis three times a week, or play pickup basketball on the weekends and maybe once during the week, you are in good shape. That isn't necessarily true, though it is better than doing nothing. But I want you to train yourself to be totally fit so that you can still maintain your regular recreational sports routine and also be in far better condition than when you started.

In so doing, I am going to ask that you make the same total commitment that I did, because without a certain sense of dedication, you simply can't achieve results. Athletes who have long careers do so, not always willingly, because they must find a way to prolong those careers. You

should wish to do so to prolong your life—and to make it happy and productive.

Dr. Kenneth Cooper, noted author on physical fitness, put matters succinctly: "Whether you live one day longer is really not the ultimate goal. What is important is the quality of your life—a life that is happy, healthy and productive."

That sort of life is a sound, makes-sense objective, and achieving it is not something that needs to be done in a kamikaze fashion.

You will not have to live for exercise. Just live better. The best way to approach this program is to set reasonable goals rather than go for broke at one time and then begin to slack off because you simply aren't able to maintain your objectives at the start. You must understand that the real effects from the training program don't really show up unless you exercise three or four times a week, but that can be done at a comfortable pace to suit your needs and goals.

How can you make this happen?

Assign specific days for the program and then make it a can't-miss part of that day's routine—at home or away. The times when you feel the least like doing it, because of pressures in your life, may be the times when you need it most to relieve stress. You probably will come out feeling like a new person. But you can't just exercise for an hour and then fall back into bad dietary habits; nor can you exercise three times a week, which is my suggested minimum, and party three days a week, too. Yes, you can have ice cream every once in a while, but don't eat a half-pint—and emphasize the "a while" in that "every once in a while."

And before you finish, you may come out looking like a new person because I also will suggest ways to complement the effects of your exercise and fitness routine in the areas of skin and hair care, nutrition and dressing that newly toned body to show it at its best.

You will be proud and pleased to keep looking as good as possible for the rest of your life. If this program does that for you, then I will have succeeded in achieving the goal I have set for myself in writing this book: getting more people to "think fit" and to "stay fit."

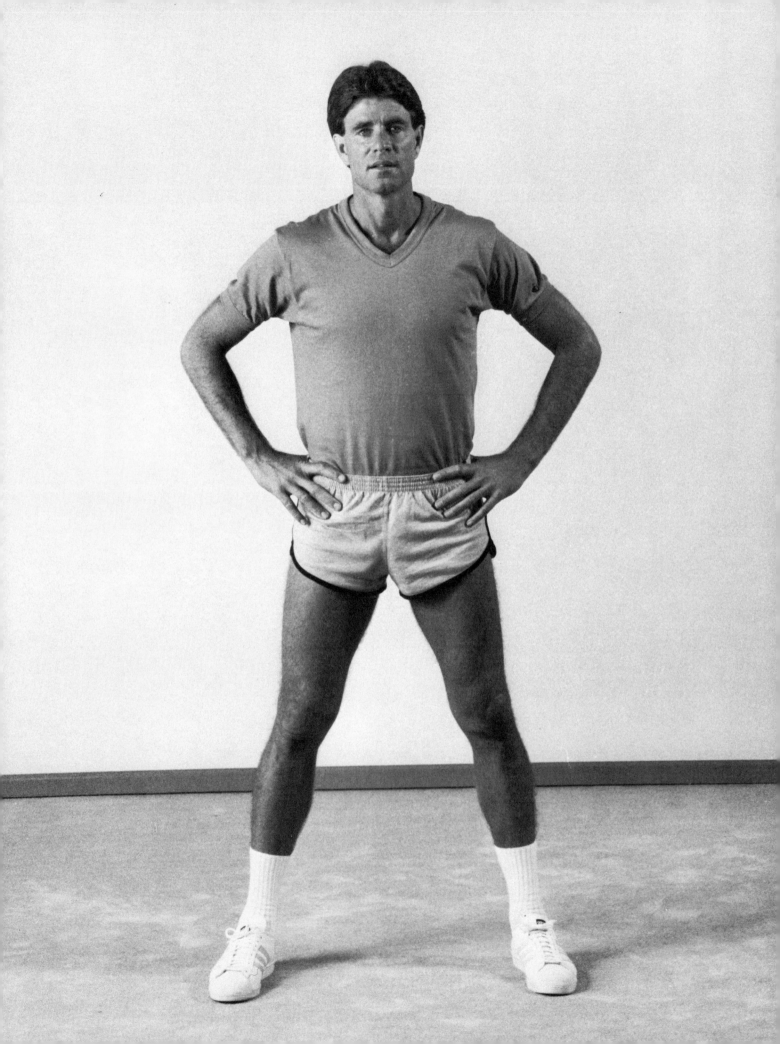

CHAPTER 2

PALMERFIT PROGRAM: LOOSENING UP, WORKING OUT, COOLING DOWN

Your body is a marvelous machine, the most precise, intricate and interesting precision instrument ever created. No one has ever been able to duplicate its parts precisely, and even replacing some of them is still a very imprecise science, in its most rudimentary stages and with no guarantee that we will ever be able to go to "the store" and order a new set of whatevers.

That, of course, means that what we have is what we always will have. It also means that we should be doing as much as any master craftsman would do in caring for a fine precision instrument—seeing that all of its working parts are properly maintained.

That is not difficult. For our body machine, if anything, it is the most natural thing in the world because our daily living takes care of so much ... moving, eating, thinking and resting, all parts of its function. However, the body usually demands more, particularly as we get older or find our lifestyle and work habits becoming more confining.

As I noted in Chapter 1, caring properly for our body means that we have to take special means over and above our daily habits. Some people simply build these means into their living routines, making them a natural part of their way of life. Most though—and you well may be one of this vast majority—have to give time and effort to doing something really extraordinary to keep their bodies in fine operating condition.

The fact that you have taken the trouble to explore some of the ideas which have been so successful for me shows that you care enough about this process to pursue it seriously. And I hope the only "serious" part of all that I will offer will be your pursuit; the rest, I hope, will be relaxing and enjoyable, and give you results that you and your body will find most pleasing.

The first part of the program is to get your body into good working order, and that is only accomplished by exercise. Oh, I know you've heard that before, but the program I am going to lay out for you is an all-encompassing method that will bring maximum satisfaction and results if you follow it to the letter ... and those letters are as easy as ABC.

I am not going to ask you to do anything that I don't do—or haven't done—myself.

First of all, I am not going to ask you to do anything that I don't do—or haven't done—myself. And I am going to give you the precise exercise routine which I have followed for years, and which not only has been effective but, more importantly, makes sense and is not harmful to your bodily well-being.

To understand exactly what you will be doing and why, let's look at some of the basic elements which comprise the overall subject of *Exercise Training.*

Exercises can be divided into the following elements:

(1) *Training Modes,* whether they are *aerobic* or *anaerobic.*

(2) *Type of movement* produced by the muscular contraction, which is *isometric, isotonic* or *isokinetic.*

Let's look at each separately.

You've heard the terms "aerobic" and "anaerobic" bandied about with a sometimes frightening glibness. Often they are used improperly to describe what may be happening to your body, or a routine that you believe may be good for you. So let's look at some very precise definitions and see how they will apply to our overall fitness program:

Aerobic Exercise: This is activity which requires the use of large amounts of oxygen over a prolonged period of time, and which will force the body, through repetitive movement, to expand its capacity to supply that oxygen. Remember, oxygen helps to fuel our muscles during exercise, and the more we can use, or can train our body to utilize, the longer we will be able to continue. In the program I shortly will lay out, we will be most concerned about expanding your aerobic capacity. Some examples of aerobic exercise are walking, jogging, running, cycling, jumping rope and swimming.

Anaerobic Exercise: Means without oxygen, which is almost the opposite of aerobic exercise. This form of exercise uses the body's store of oxygen faster than it can be replaced. Exercises of this type demand such enormous amounts of oxygen that they can only be done for a short period of time.

Here are two examples which illustrate the differences between aerobic and anaerobic exercises. Someone running a marathon is performing aerobic exercise because his form of exercise is consuming oxygen at a rate that permits him to continue over a long period of time, and he has trained to increase the consumption from the time he first began jogging, to the point where he now can run nonstop for more than 26 miles.

Someone running the 100-yard dash is performing *anaerobic exercise* because for no more than 10 seconds or so he is requiring his body to supply enough oxygen to get through that particular race.

The training benefits of aerobic exercise are many. Certainly, through regular training you should be able to lower your resting heart rate, which means the heart will not be beating as fast or working as hard at rest. Thus, you can sustain work, or exercise, for long periods; your heart becomes more efficient, assuring a steady supply of blood and oxygen to all organs and limbs; and your entire muscle system is more efficiently "fed" by an increased supply of oxygen.

One of the best living examples of someone who had great aerobic capacity is John Havlicek.

One of the best living examples of someone who had great aerobic capacity is John Havlicek, the former basketball player for the Boston Celtics, who, when he finally retired after seventeen seasons, had played more games and more minutes than anyone in pro basketball history. John was famous for his great endurance on the court, in a sport that requires nearly non-stop

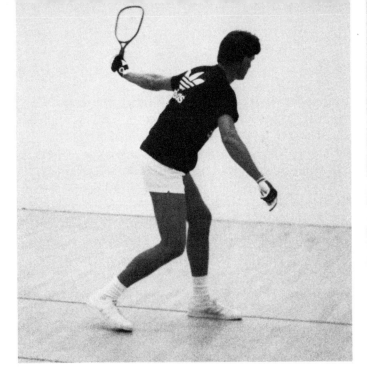
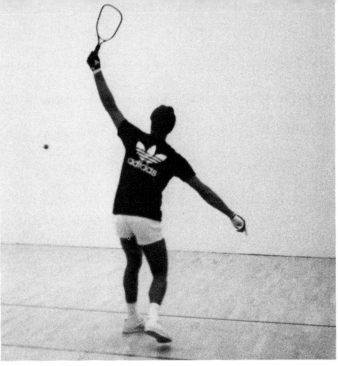

movement. He never seemed to tire, and you could see him forcefully urging younger teammates to more effort during crucial games simply by running past them and giving them a nudge or a word of encouragement. To have played thousands of games and tens of thousands of minutes over so many years was remarkable. But there was a very good reason why John could do it.

Those who knew John, such as pitcher Phil Niekro, one of his childhood friends, have often said that he unconsciously trained himself for such endurance because as a boy he ran everywhere—to the store, to school, to the playground, on the playground. Phil has said John was a perpetual-motion machine, never content to walk but always running. "He must have a pair of bellows [lungs] that could have fired a steel furnace" is how Phil put it, and he should know since he was raised in an Ohio steel town.

We are not going to train you aerobically to be John Havlicek or give you a routine that is made only for those in professional sports. However, many non-athletes have discovered great aerobic potential when enrolled in an exercise program. What follows will be a routine that anyone—athlete and non-athlete alike—can do. I did it to help my baseball skills; you can do it to help whatever physical attributes or skills you may wish to pursue.

Now for the three various types of movement which are produced by muscular contraction:

(1) *Isometric Exercise:* This contracts muscles without moving any joints or extremities. Examples include contracting your muscles in the abdomen, arms, legs, or pushing against a standing object for 5 to 10 seconds before relaxing them. The process then is repeated, and it can be done at your desk, while driving your car, walking down the street—anyplace.

There will be no quick, dramatic results, and if anything, these may be best characterized as "maintenance exercises." Heart specialists, however, have frowned on cardiac patients pursuing exercises of this type because that sudden gripping could cause a dangerous rise in blood pressure. Remember not to hold your breath while doing them.

(2) *Isotonic Exercise:* This involves the contraction of a muscle with concurrent movements of a joint over the full range of motion. Calisthenics and weight lifting are examples.

(3) *Isokinetic Exercise:* This means moving the muscles against continuous pressure, and is used in the evaluation of muscular strength.

Virtually all the muscles of the body will come into play as we pursue our program and they will be self-evident.

While I have done various types of exercises over the years, the unique feature of this program is that we will be training aerobically and isotonically through sports as well as through exercise.

Every exercise program has three distinct phases:

(1) *Warm Up:* This consists of first increasing the muscle temperature and slowly increasing the heart rate for the activity that is to come; followed by about 12 to 15 minutes of stretching the muscles that will be involved in the exercise program.

(2) *Workout:* A specific number of movements which will affect the body as a whole. You cannot exercise for "spot" weight reduction (which we will discuss later), but an overall program, in concert with other actions, can achieve that end. After the specific exercises, there is about a 20-minute period or longer, if you wish, for your own choice of aerobic physical activity, such as jogging or stationary bike riding.

(3) *Cooldown:* A repeat of the stretching exercises while the muscles still are warm that will help return respiration and heart rate to a pre-exercise rate and equalize the blood flow to all parts of the body.

Before beginning, there are a few checks to make so that you will be more comfortable and thus be able to get the most from your work:

(1) Don't eat for approximately 2 hours before exercising. Now, I'm talking about a heavy meal that fills you, not a light snack that might provide a quick energy lift. I'll often grab an apple or granola bar on the way out of the house, but I'd never come away from lunch or supper and go all-out for an hour's exercise. When I pitched for the Orioles, I always ate my pre-game meal at least 4 hours before the game's start, something that is standard for all professional sports.

(2) Attempt to keep your fluid intake minimal prior to stretching, and void just prior to beginning the program. You can replenish fluids during and after you have completed the program, and you will certainly be more comfortable moving around if you don't feel bloated or full. However, when doing aerobic exercise, don't wait till you're thirsty. Replenish fluids often.

(3) Be aware of your body to recognize whether all parts are in smooth working order. Be particularly aware of pain in a particular area, and if you are unsure of its cause, seek an answer from someone who really knows. Pain is nature's way of telling your body that something may be wrong;

a specialist will let you know what it is and whether it presents a current or potential problem to your playing routine.

(4) Be aware of how you look after exercising for a period of time and see if you notice any changes in how your body feels and looks.

(5) Use the proper attire. The key is to wear what will be comfortable and healthy and appropriate to weather conditions. Light colors reflect heat; dark ones absorb it. Be sure your shoes give your feet good support, and provide for shock absorption with a good, cushioned rubber sole.

WARMUP

Before we even begin what is commonly known as "exercise," we must treat our body like a fine automobile engine. Those who care for their cars never step into one that has been sitting overnight, or for a long period of time, and drive right off. They first allow the engine to warm up, and, indeed, most cars now have a system that will automatically rev an engine to a point where the engine itself signifies it is ready, by decreasing its revolutions per minute.

Our body demands the same treatment—a warmup and stretching phase, so that all of our parts will be properly prepared for more strenuous activity. I can vouch for the necessity of such a program by an awkward accident that I had at my own home.

I jumped out of bed one morning several years ago and decided on the moment that my lawn needed cutting. Stopping only to don a pair of athletic shorts and sneakers, I rolled out my mower and began the job. I mostly guided that mower up and down an incline and did so with total disdain until ... until I felt a stab of pain behind my right leg. I had learned enough about the body and its components to know almost immediately that I had a serious problem with my Achilles' tendon.

An examination showed that I had over-stretched it—a bit more stretch and it could have ruptured—and that accident put me out of action for several weeks. That was serious, but my own carelessness—and that is all I can call it—hurt even more. I knew—and, indeed, had practiced

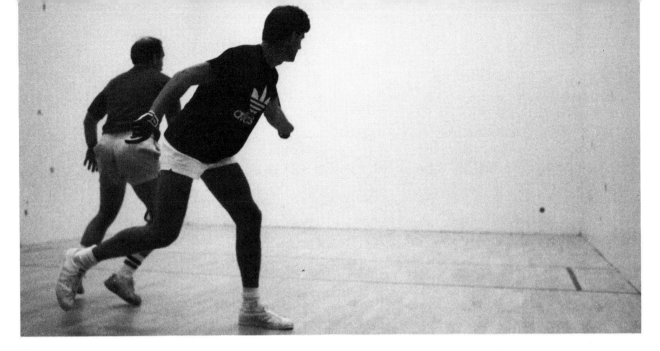

almost religiously—that whenever I was about to do any kind of physical activity, even something as simple as cutting the lawn, I had to do some kind of stretching to prepare my muscles. In fact, every time I walked out of the dugout to pitch, I stopped and stretched my legs on the dugout steps, even though I might already have pitched seven or eight innings. But that morning, for some reason, I let the habit fly past.

The First Commandment always must be: Warm up.

So the First Commandment always must be: Warm up, whether you are a superbly conditioned athlete or work in a sedentary job. Not only will it guard against cramps, strains, sprains and pulled Achilles' tendons, but it also will guarantee your heart a smooth transition into some brisk activity, and improve your performance.

This is particularly true if you are over thirty five, because your heart, like that car engine, cannot go from full rest to stressful activity without a warmup. And if you are over thirty five, be certain to get a physical examination before undergoing any program so there will be no problems.

A warmup routine has two components: *cardiovascular* and *muscular-skeletal.* Each is important, and neither can be ignored.

The *cardiovascular* component can be as simple as marching in place or walking ... anything to rouse the heart from its passive state and alert it to get ready for some action. Three minutes of marching in place, beginning slowly and then lifting the knees higher and higher, will raise your muscle temperature so you can begin your stretching exercises. Some even have advised riding a stationary bike and pedaling easily for 3 to 5 minutes. If you wish, begin by marching in place for a couple of minutes and then get on the bike and complete the process.

Stretching

Stretching is the next step in warming up the muscles. I can think of no more important models in this regard than the stretching routines of sports teams. Years ago, teams would spread themselves across a practice field and do 10 or 15 minutes of calisthenics, and then go about their practice routines.

Now, savvy teams emphasize stretching more than those old exercise routines because they expect their athletes to be in shape when they report for training, and they understand the necessity of having muscles as supple and flexible as possible before beginning any hard work. The routines now have been extended to the same ones which we will follow—stretching before and at the end of practice to help the cooldown process. If it is worthy of a team that is trying to protect millions of dollars' worth of playing talent, then it certainly is worthy of your efforts.

How you stretch is every bit as important as why you do it. Here are some very good guidelines:

(1) Don't stretch too far, especially in the beginning—just a gentle, slight stretch so that you feel some pull in the muscle. If it begins to hurt, ease off a bit.

(2) Hold the stretch in a comfortable position for about 20 seconds. Relax and stretch again. As your flexibility increases, work up to 30 seconds.

(3) Don't bob or bounce because you could tear muscle fibers and injure yourself.

(4) Breathe slowly and naturally and do not hold your breath. Establish a rhythm: Exhale as you perform the positive movement and inhale as you perform the negative movement (return to starting position).

One last item before beginning the program is to take your *Resting Heart Rate,* which really means taking your own pulse. You can do this in any one of three ways—place your hand over your heart and count the number of beats; place your finger on your windpipe at the neck and move it to the groove on

either side; or place your middle finger on the inside of your wrist at the base of your thumb and move it about an inch up your forearm. Count the beats for 10 seconds and then multiply that number by 6, which gives you a heart rate for one minute. That is your Resting Heart Rate, and it will become a point of reference in measuring your improvement in aerobic capacity as you continue this program.

As that capacity improves, the Resting Heart Rate will diminish because the heart will become more efficient and stronger in its capacity to pump blood throughout your system.

Here are the flexibility or stretching exercises, the initial phase of the program:

(1) *Neck Bends:* Standing with feet at shoulder width and hands on hips, slowly lower your head onto your chest, hold 10 seconds and return to straight position. Next, move it backward as far as possible and hold for 10 seconds, before returning to straight position. Then lower head to left shoulder, hold 10 seconds and return to straight position. Do the same toward right shoulder and hold for same time before returning. This stretches most of the neck muscles.

(2) *Twister:* Standing with feet at shoulder width, arms at sides and slightly away from body, rotate head, then trunk, clockwise so that you are

Neck Bends

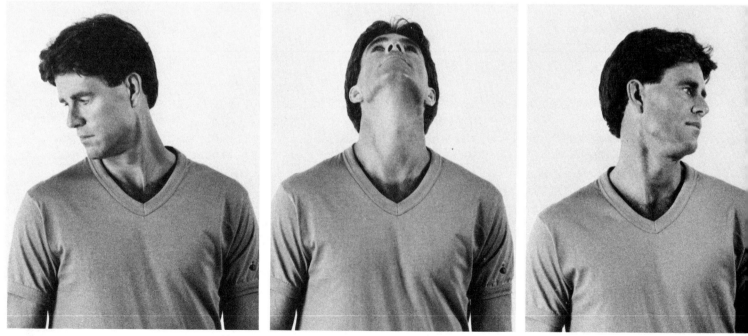

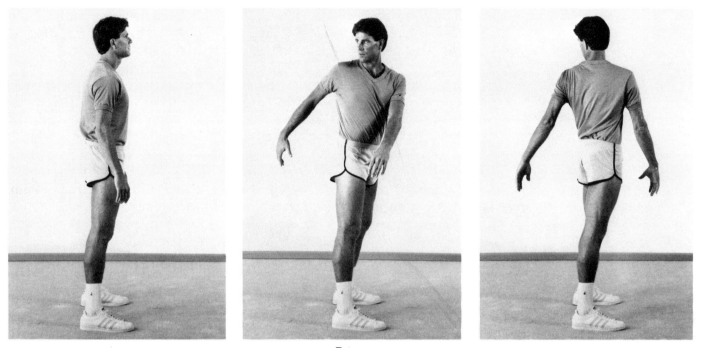

Twister

looking over your right shoulder at your heels. Lead with head and allow arms to help pull you around. Return to starting position, then do same move to left. Do alternately 2 times each, holding each stretch for 20 seconds. This stretches abdominal and back muscles.

(3) *Side Bends:* Feet at shoulder width and a towel held with both hands in front. Lift towel over head and, from waist, bend to right and hold for 5 seconds; return to upright position and bring towel back down to front. Repeat towel raise and bend to the left, holding 5 seconds, and return to starting position. Alternate each direction 5 times. This stretches some abdominal and back muscles which bend you to the side.

(4) *Overhead Stretch:* Feet at shoulder width and a towel held in front with both hands. Very slowly raise arms and towel over head and behind body, then return to starting position. Entire circular motion is done 5 times to count of 10 to stretch the muscles which elevate and rotate the arms.

(5) *Airplane Stretch:* Feet at shoulder width and towel again held in front. Without bending trunk, lift arms over head and move them far enough to right so that left arm is above head. Hold for 5 count. Alternate to left side and do each direction 5 times to stretch muscles beneath shoulder and along rib cage.

(6) *Two-Arm Hug and Reverse Two-Arm Hug:* Feet at shoulder width with arms raised in front at 90 degrees to your body. Cross right arm over to touch left shoulder, and left arm to touch right shoulder; pull as if to hug yourself. Hold 20 seconds to stretch muscles behind your shoulder and upper back. Do 2 times. For *Reverse Two-Arm Hug,* start at same position, bend elbow 90 degrees, pull arms behind body, pinching shoulder blades together. Hold 20 seconds.

(7) *Groin Stretch:* Start upright with feet spread at shoulder width. Move right foot 2 feet to the side, then shift body weight to right leg, bending right hip and knee while keeping left knee straight. Keep toes pointed straight ahead and feel stretch inside left thigh as you hold the position for 20 seconds. Reverse the action to the left and do each 2 times to stretch groin muscles and those inside thigh.

(8) *Sprinter:* Start at same position as Groin Stretch, with feet 4 feet apart. Rotate to the right on balls of feet so that you and your feet are facing sideways. Lean forward on right foot by bending right hip and knee, and keep the left leg straight with the weight on the ball of your foot to feel a stretch in front of left hip. Hold the position 20 seconds, then return to upright position. Do this 2

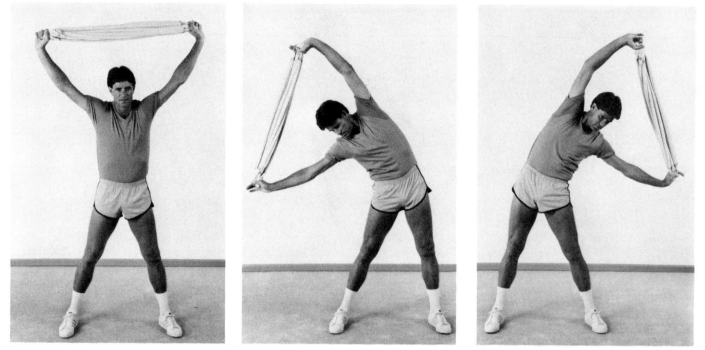

Side Bends

Overhead Stretch

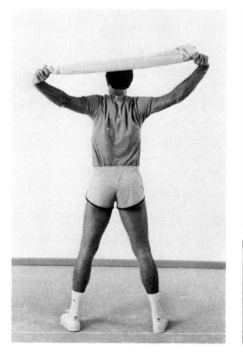
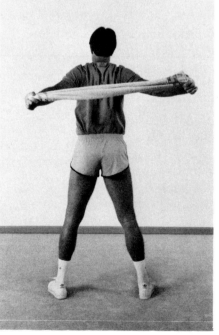
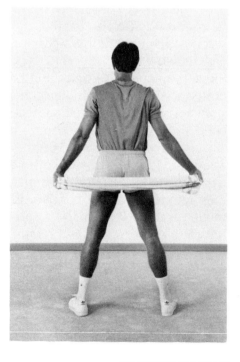

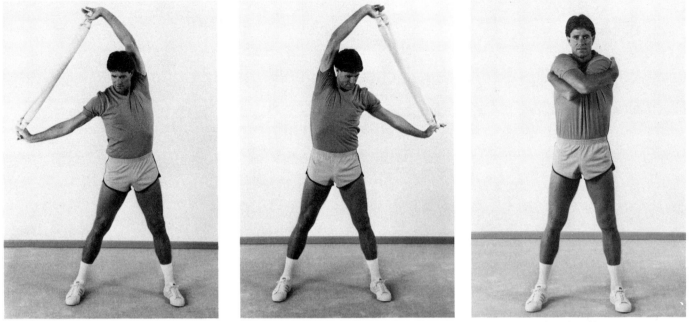

Windmill or Airplane Stretch

Two-Arm Hug

Reverse Two-Arm Hug

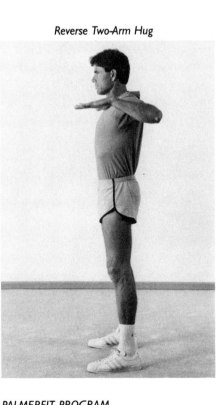

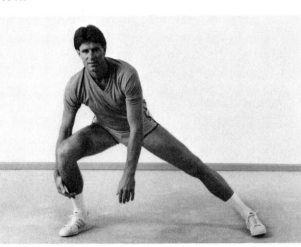

Groin Stretch

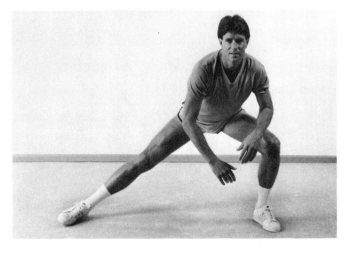

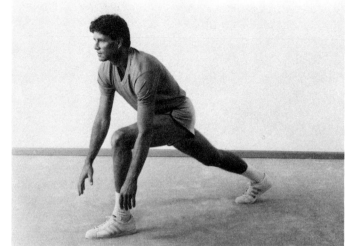

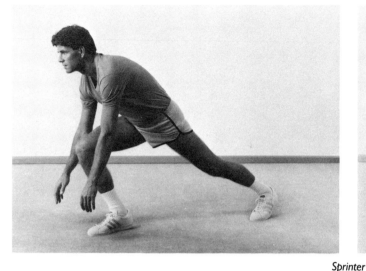

Sprinter

times to the right, then 2 times to left, to stretch the muscles in front of the hip.

(9) *Parallel Leg Stretch:* Feet at shoulder width, bend right knee and raise right heel to your buttocks. Grasp right leg just above the ankle and pull backward, keeping it parallel to the left leg and not allowing it to swing outward. It is okay to use a standing object for balance. Hold the position 20 seconds and perform 2 times alternately. For an even greater stretch, lean body forward and *attempt* to pull leg parallel to floor.

Quad or Parallel Leg Stretch

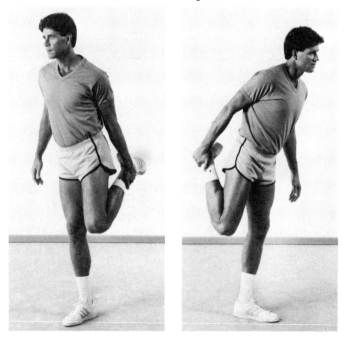

(10) *Achilles' Tendon or Heel Cord Stretch:* Stand at least 4 feet from a wall or eye-level standing object with both feet even and about a foot apart. Lift arms to shoulder level, keeping heels flat on floor, and lean forward from ankles with elbows bent, touching wall or standing object with your palms to feel stretch in your calf. Hold for 20 seconds and do 2 times to stretch your calf muscle. Toes and feet must be pointed straight ahead.

With *no wall or standing object* for balance, stand with one leg in front of the other, bend right hip and knee so you are leaning forward onto it. Maintain back, or left, leg with knee straight and heel down, to stretch that calf muscle. Hold 20 seconds and do alternately 2 times.

The next exercises can be done from a sitting position:

Achilles' Tendon Stretch

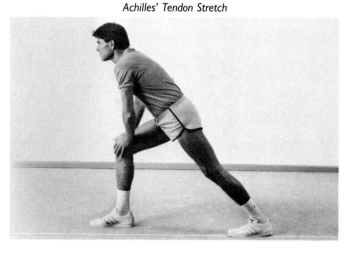

(11) *Hamstring Stretch:* Seated on floor with legs straight, bend forward, knees straight, and attempt to touch toes. If you cannot straighten knees, forget about touching toes and concentrate instead on keeping legs straight by pushing them down onto the floor. Either way, be certain to stretch forward and curl forward to touch your toes, holding the stretch 20 seconds. Exhale while attempting to touch forward. Do 2 times.

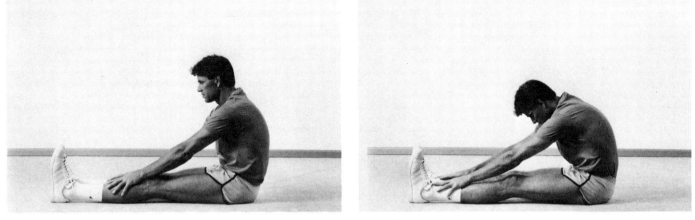

Hamstring Stretching/Knees Straight

Hamstring Stretching/Spread Legs 4 ft. Apart

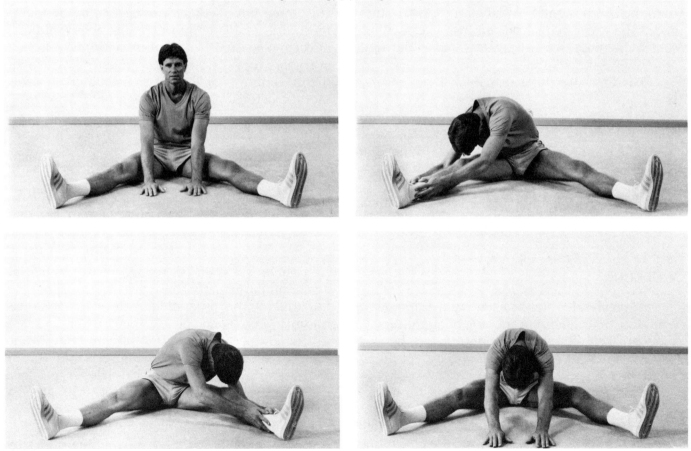

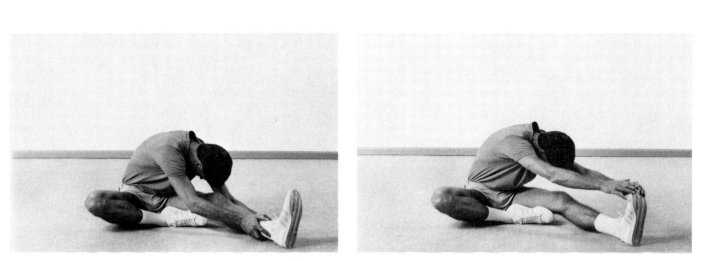

Hamstring Stretching/Single-Leg Stretch

(12) *Hurdler:* Sit in a straddle position with legs approximately 3 to 4 feet apart. Bend the right leg at the knee so the right ankle crosses just above the left knee. Push down at the right knee to stretch, and hold 20 seconds before releasing. Do this 2 times, then switch to the *Reverse Hurdler* with the bent leg behind your body. Attempt to lean back and away from the bent leg and hold 20 seconds. Do 2 times, and then switch to right side for both exercises, to stretch the muscles which rotate the thigh outward and straighten the knee.

The final stretching exercise is done *lying on your back.*

(13) *Back Stretch:* Bend your right hip and knee and grasp back of thigh and pull it to your chest, holding 20 seconds and then releasing. Do not allow back to come too far off floor. Repeat with left leg for same time. When finished, bring both legs together on chest and hold at the back of the thigh, just below knees, for 20 seconds. Do each leg 2 times, then both legs 2 times.

WORKOUT

Your muscles and heart are tuned up and ready for the exercise or training phase of the program. And if you are just starting out, be reasonable about your goals. If you cannot do all of the recommended repetitions, don't worry about it. The idea really is to finish the program, and you cannot reasonably expect to step into something like this after a long period of inactivity and go through it easily. Don't burn yourself out

on the first half of the program and be unable to continue. Your muscles will tell you, as you do each repetition, just how much they have left. When there is fatigue, stop and go on to the next exercise.

At the end of this chapter there is a Workout Chart, page 33, that lists, by your degree of fitness (Beginner, Intermediate, Advanced), the number of repetitions and length of time for each repetition of each exercise. I have constructed this to help everyone, regardless of his experience level, to gain the maximum benefit so as to be able to go right into the aerobic phase of the workout when the exercises are finished and still be capable of gaining the maximum benefit from both phases.

There is no specific exercise that will help to shrink a particular portion of your body.

There is one other area which you should be aware of, particularly those of you who are undertaking this program as part of a weight-loss routine. There is no specific exercise that will help to shrink a particular portion of your body. Some claim that when you feel the muscles in that flabby area begin to pinch or burn, you have begun to work on that specific area. Not true—you are toning the muscles, but you are not necessarily burning fat. Those are only signs that the muscle is getting fatigued because it is not getting sufficient

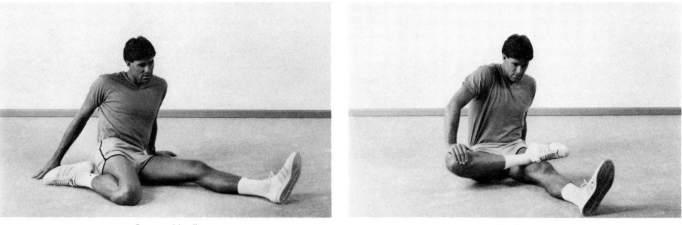

Reverse Hurdler   Hurdler

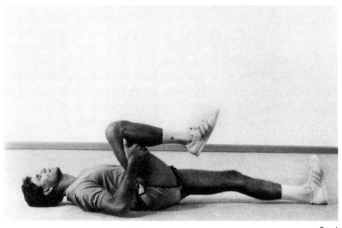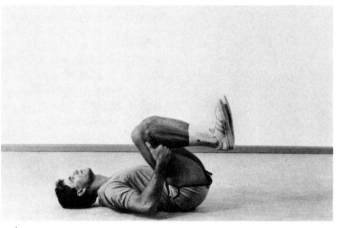

Back Stretch

oxygen to continue. That's why I advised earlier to back off, give that muscle a break to help it to renew its oxygen supply, and then continue your exercises. A balanced program, helped by a balanced diet, will soon begin to work off your excess poundage in a way that will give your body an overall tone. The best weight-loss routine really is a pushaway—push away from the table before you consume too much food. Coupling it with exercise will provide for a balanced and even loss.

In fact, most people find that exercise cuts down their appetite. Many think that the more you exercise or are active, the hungrier you will get, but just the opposite is true. So don't get hung up on the simple weight-loss routine; stay with the program and you will begin to see the difference, both in your body profile and in your reduced need for food.

We'll now go to our exercises, but remember that they will be done at optimum levels, which are found on the accompanying Workout Chart, page 33. If you are just beginning, or have been away from a regular exercise program for some time, begin with the low number of repetitions. If you exercise regularly, you can begin with the intermediate levels; and if you are advanced, start with the highest level. And don't worry about performing different exercises at different levels of difficulty. Meet your own capabilities.

You finished your warmup or stretching exercises lying on your back, so you will now begin the exercise program from the same position, making the continuity much more natural and not interrupting your flow or bodily rhythm.

(1) *Pelvic Tilt:* Lying on your back with hips and knees slightly bent, roll the pelvis backward so that your back is flattened on the floor. In that position, hold for 5 seconds. Repeat 10 times.

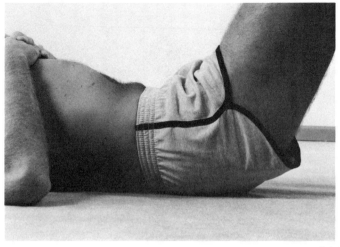
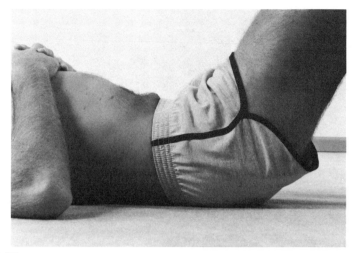

Pelvic Tilt

(2) *Partial Sit-up or Crunches:* Lying on floor with hips and knees slightly bent, do a pelvic tilt and curl your head 8 to 10 inches off floor and up on your chest. Hold 5 seconds and curl back to starting position. *Do not arch your back.* Exhale and repeat 10 times.

(3) *Full Sit-up:* Lying on floor with hips and knees slightly bent, do a pelvic tilt and curl upper body to full sitting position, again not arching the back. This can be done with arms and hands at the side, folded across chest or clasped on forehead. Hold 5 seconds and roll back to starting position. Repeat 10 times. *A note of caution:* In order to reduce cheating, and lessen chance for injury, initiate all sit-up exercises with head and shoulder curl. If the sit-up is done incorrectly, the abdominal muscles will not be working. If the back is arched when doing a sit-up, the hip muscles are being used and the abdominal muscles are being stretched and strained; and if momentum is used to aid the sit-up, then the appropriate muscles are not properly used. Do not have your feet held down by another person or inanimate object because the hip muscles will work instead of the abdominals.

(4) *Bent Knee-up or Partial Leg Lowering:* Lying on back legs extended, with hands on abdomen below ribs, and keeping small of back in contact with floor, bring one leg up so hip is flexed beyond 90 degrees, with knee bent freely downward. Bring other leg to same position, but still keep back flat on floor, and place hands just below ribs. If abdomen is not tightening, you are doing this incorrectly. Hold final position for 20 seconds and return feet to floor.

Partial Sit-up

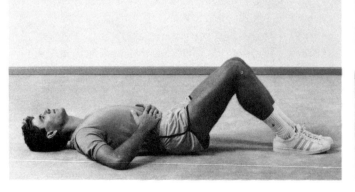
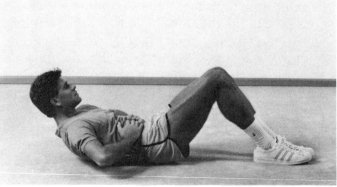

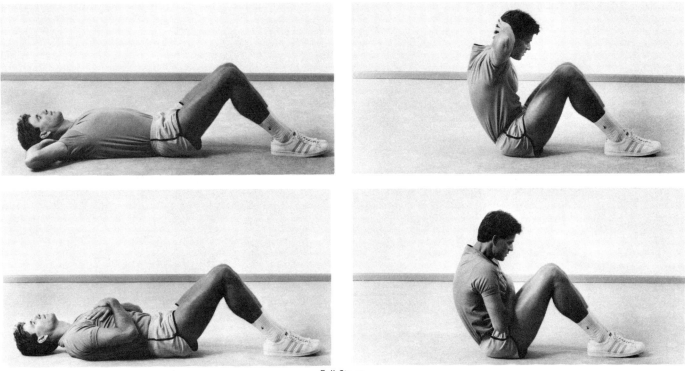

Full Sit-up

Bent Knee-up or Partial Leg Lowering

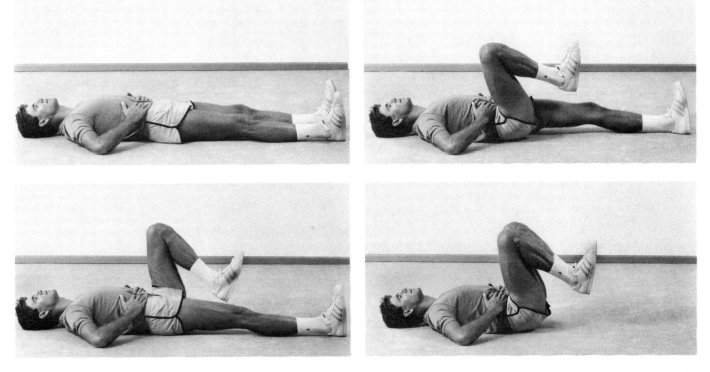

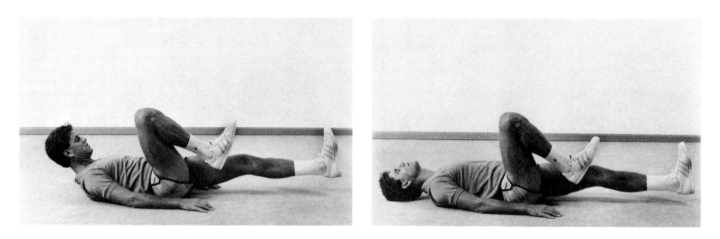

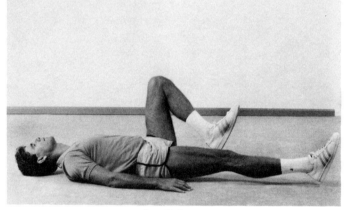

Bow & Arrow

(5) *Bow and Arrow:* Lying on back, bend one leg so hip is flexed at 90 degrees and other leg is straight out. Push flexed leg to straight-leg position while bringing straight one back to flexed state.

(6) *Rollover:* Lying on back with knees straight, bring left leg to 90-degree flex and move it across body toward right hip, attempting to touch toe to floor. Keep hip and shoulders flat on floor. Return leg to straight position and back on floor. For *Reverse Rollover,* flex leg to 90 degrees and move it to side; bring it back to 90-degree flex, and return to straight-leg position on floor. Repeat with opposite leg.

(7) *Barbell Arms:* Lying on floor with arms at sides and palms facing upward, bend elbow to touch shoulder.

(8) *Paddle Arms:* Lie on back with knees bent and feet flat on floor. Bend elbow to 90 degrees. Place one arm at 90 degrees to trunk so back of hand touches floor, and rotate other arm forward so palm touches floor. Keep arms at 90 degrees and alternate arm movements.

(9) *Punch Up Arms:* Lying on back with arms extended to the sides, bend arms at elbows so lower arms are at 90 degrees to upperarms and parallel to trunk, with hand touching floor behind head. Straighten elbow with upward punching motion. Alternate each arm.

Note: Consult Workout Chart notes for maximum workout benefits using weights for exercises 7–9 listed on page 33.

(10) *Side Leg Lift:* Lying on side with body in straight line, bend bottom leg 90 degrees at the knee. Place top arm in front and bottom one in straight line with body, above head. Lift upper leg as high as possible toward ceiling, slightly behind pelvis, with foot also pointed slightly upward, and return to original position. Do not allow leg to go to front of pelvis while being lifted.

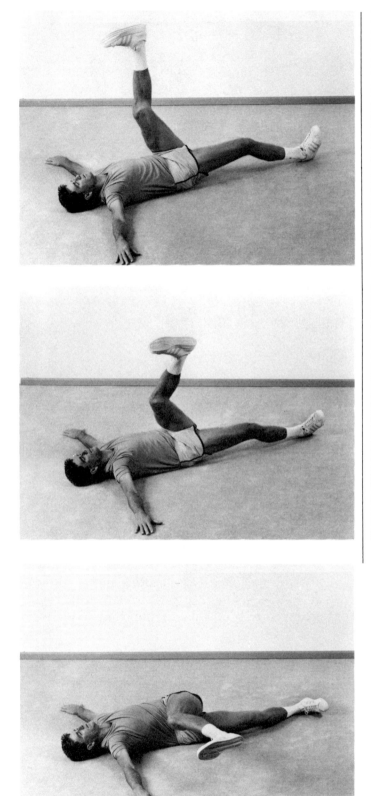

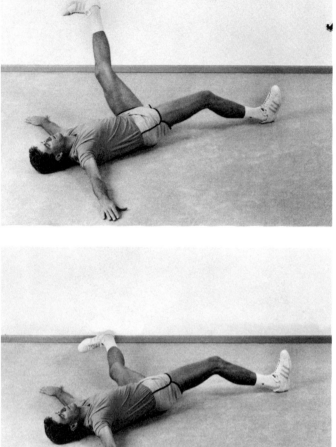

Reverse Rollover

(11) *Reverse Leg Lift:* Sitting with hands to the side and rear, bend upper leg in front of body with foot resting flat on floor. Lift underneath leg toward ceiling, with knee pointed forward and return to original position. A variation is to place legs together and lift toward ceiling.

(12) *Back Leg Lift—Bent Knee:* Lie face down on floor and bend right knee 90 degrees. Lift right leg slightly off floor by contracting buttocks. Do not roll onto opposite hip, and keep abdomen and pelvis flat on floor.

(13) *Back Leg Lift—Straight Knee:* Lie face down on floor with both legs straight and lift right leg slightly off floor from the hip. Lift 10 times and repeat with opposite leg.

Rollover

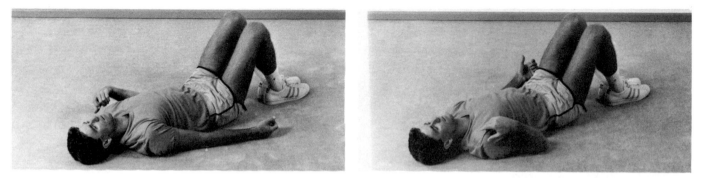

Barbell Arms

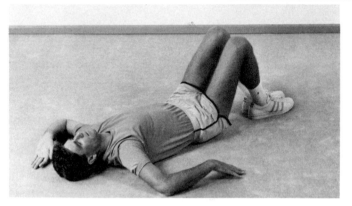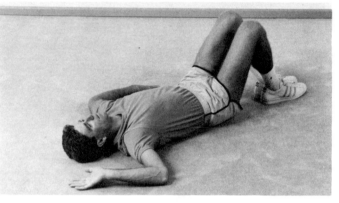

Paddle Arms

Punch Up Arms

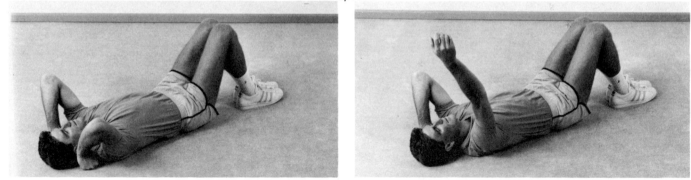

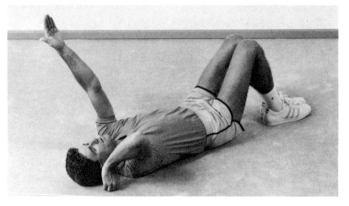

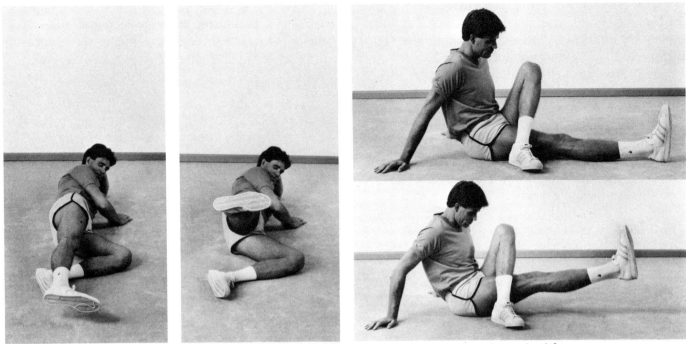

Side Leg Lift

Reverse Leg Lift

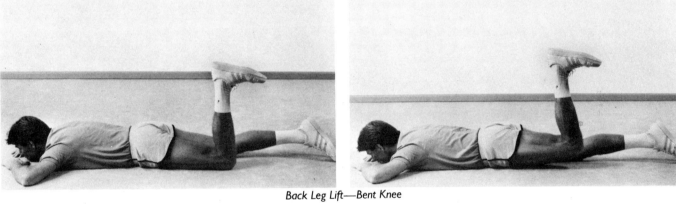

Back Leg Lift—Bent Knee

Back Leg Lift—Straight Knee

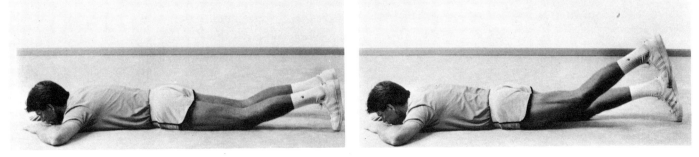

(14) *Back Lift:* Lying on floor face down, keep arms next to body, with palms facing out. Lift both arms back and slowly lift head, neck and upper back from floor, holding that position.

(15) *Push-up:* Lying face down on floor, arms bent, hands facing forward, under or just outside shoulders, push up, keeping body straight. Rest weight on toes and hands. Do not allow midsection to sag or butt to rise past body line. Dip back to floor in straight-line position and push upward again.

(16) *Arm Circle:* Stand with feet at shoulder width and arms straight out at 90 degrees from shoulder. Rotate arm in small circles forward with palm facing down. For *Reverse Arm Circle,* change direction and rotate arms to rear, with palms upward. Make circles approximately 12 inches.

(17) *Juggle Arms:* Stand with feet at shoulder width, with both arms 90 degrees to front of body, palms downward and elbows straight. Raise one arm overhead while dropping other to side. Alternate arms.

(18) *Windmill Arms:* Standing with feet at shoulder width, lift right arm to ear, keeping left at side. Lower elevated arm to side and lift other at same time to elevated position, keeping both elbows straight.

(19) *Side Bend:* Standing with feet at shoulder width and arms at 90 degrees to side of body, bend body sideward without rotating forward or backward and, with knees slightly flexed, slowly reach toward ankle.

Back Lift   *Push-up*

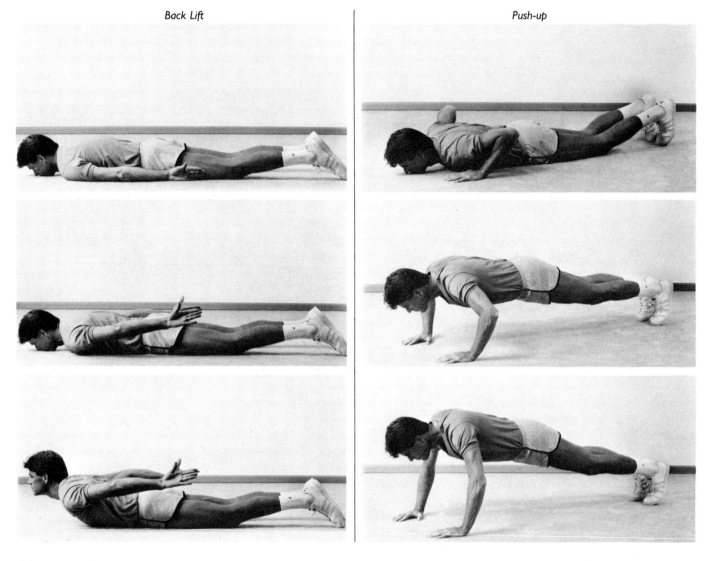

Arm Circle   *Reverse Arm Circle*   *Juggle Arms*

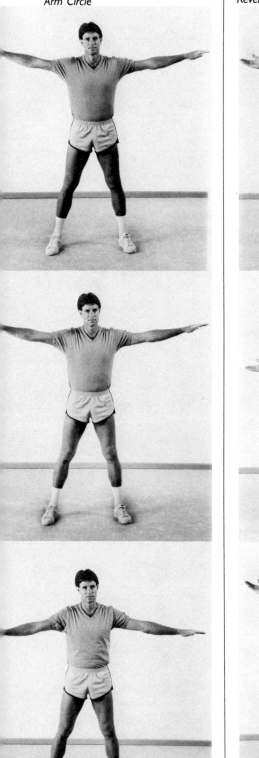

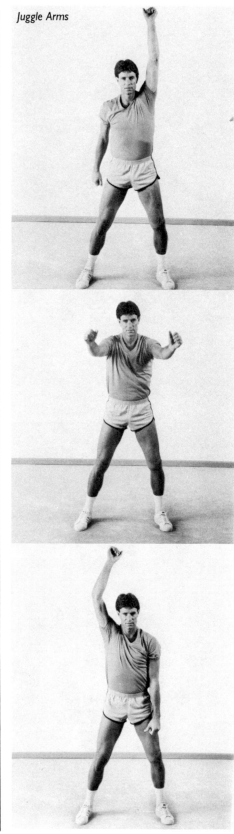

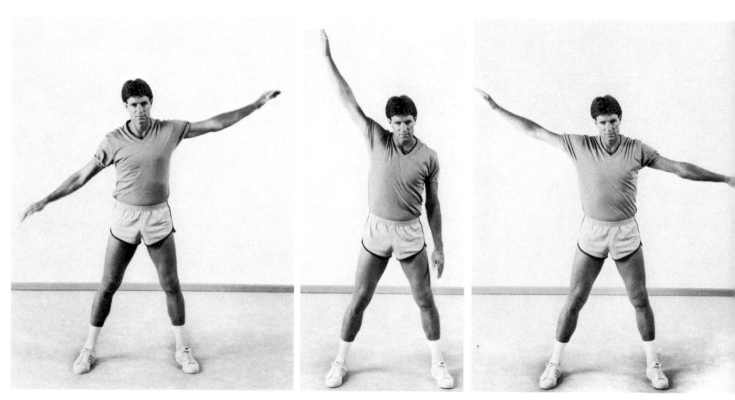

Windmill Arms

Side Bend

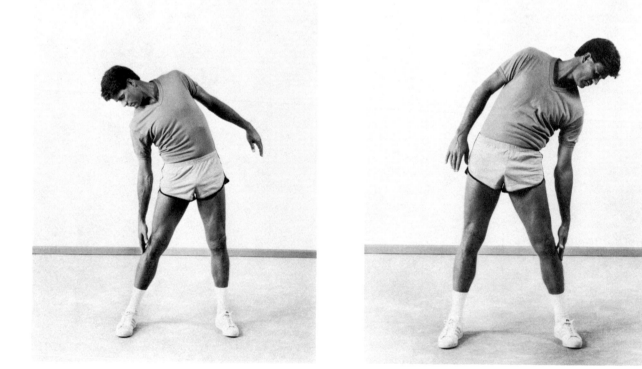

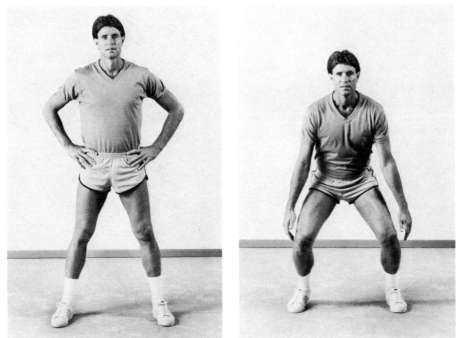

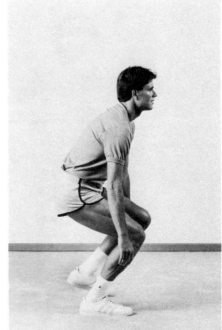

Double Leg Half-Squat

Single Leg Half-Squat

(20) *Double-Leg Half-Squat:* Standing with feet 2 to 3 feet apart, squat to bend at hips and knees, but with back straight. *Do not go all the way down.*

(21) *Single-Leg Half-Squat:* Standing with legs 2 to 3 feet apart, lift one leg behind your body to 90 degrees and bend opposite hip and knee to squat position, lowering body to 45 degrees. *Do not go all the way down.* Keep your trunk forward to balance weight on lifted leg. When beginning this exercise, you may wish to support yourself with the opposite arm.

(22) *Heel Raise:* Standing with legs 2 to 3 feet apart, lift one leg from floor with knees bent behind your body, placing all your weight on firm leg. Raise up on ball of foot and return to foot-flat position.

(23) *Biceps Raise:* Standing with feet about a foot apart, wrap an elastic band, cut from an old inner tube or a piece of medical tubing, around your foot; bend from the trunk to grasp it, return to upright position and curl it upward toward your shoulder. Then return to original position.

There are two additional exercises, each done from the supine (lying on back) position, which can be used by those who are in the advanced category. The first, called the (3A) *V Sit-up,* can be done after the Full Sit-up, from a semi-reclining position with trunk at 45-degree angle to knees and

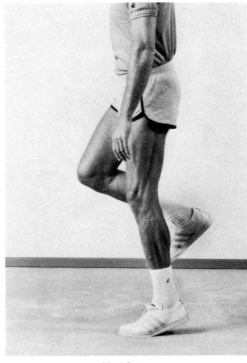

Heel Raise

hips at the same angle. Move trunk and legs toward each other to make a V, and then partially extend them. Move trunk toward lying position and push legs to straightened position, toward floor, and bring both feet together.

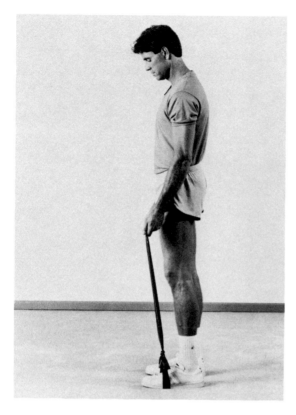 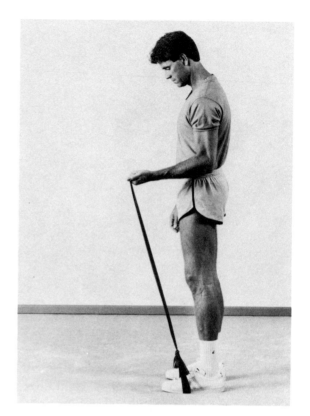

Biceps Raise

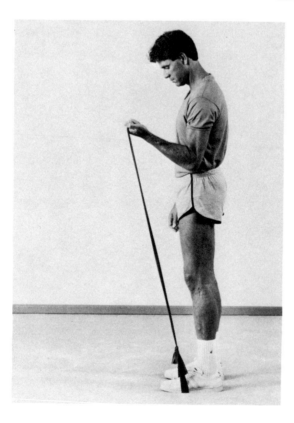 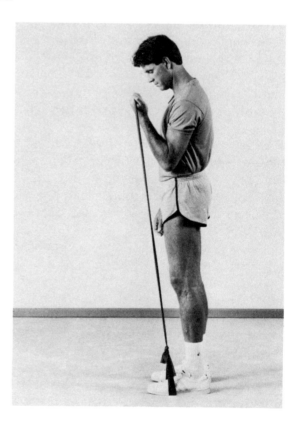

The other is a (5A) *Double-Leg Lowering Lift,* performed after the Bow & Arrow. Do a pelvic tilt, and, lying on back, lift both legs upward to 90 degrees with feet pointed toward ceiling. Slowly lower them to floor, maintaining a flat back. If back starts to arch while lowering the legs, stop this exercise.

AEROBIC EXERCISE ACTIVITY

Once you have finished the exercise program, your real work lies ahead because you have prepared yourself for a minimum of 20 minutes of brisk aerobic exercise activity. A word of caution: If you're just beginning after years of neglect, start slowly with as few as 5 to 10 minutes and work up to the 20-minute minimum. These activities can include jogging in place, walking, fast walking, rope jumping, stationary rowing, stationary cycling, jogging forward, backward and to the side from an in-place position, and stair climbing.

You also must monitor your heartbeat during this activity, starting with the end of the exercise program. First you must know two things: your *Maximum Heart Rate* and your *Target Heart Rate.*

Your Maximum Heart Rate is determined by taking your pulse for 10 seconds and then multiplying the number of beats by 6. This will give the number of heartbeats per minute. Seventy-two is average. Take your pulse midway through your aerobic exercise activity. Next, subtract your age from 220. At 40 years of age, an individual's maximum heart rate would be 220 minus 40, or 180.

To find your Target Heart Rate, take 60 percent of that Maximum Heart Rate figure. In this case, 60 percent of 180 is 108. If your heart exceeds that figure during your aerobic exercise workout, you are training too hard. Trained athletes may determine their Target Heart Rate by multiplying their Maximum Heart Rate by 80 percent. For a 40-year-old athlete, the Target Heart Rate would be 144 beats per minute. If you can train continuously at your Target Heart Rate for 20 minutes or more, you will improve your fitness and expand your aerobic capacity—that is, your heart will be able to do more work more efficiently.

COOLDOWN EXERCISES

With the muscles in your body warm from all of your activity, this is the perfect time for some stretching because the muscles will react smoothly to your routine—and that routine is the same as the one which began your program. In other words, just go back and repeat your original stretching exercises until your breathing returns to a pre-exercise level.

I have prepared a frequency chart that will indicate just how often you should do these routines and then couple them with the sports activities and their allied exercises which I will discuss in the following chapter.

WARMUP CHART
JIM PALMER FLEXIBILITY FITNESS EXERCISES
F/AE (Flexibility/Aerobic Exercise)

POSITION	WARMUP/STRETCHING		*MINIMUM HOLD TIME
	3-MIN JOG IN PLACE, WALK, SLOW STATIONARY BIKE		
Standing Position	1 Neck Bend	Alternate 2X each way—right/left, front/back	10 count each
	2 Twister	Alternate 2X each way—right/left	20 sec. hold
	3 Side Bend (with towel)	5X one way—right, 5X other way—left	5 sec. hold
	4 Overhead Stretch (with towel)	Alternate 5X each way—front/back	10 count
	5 Airplane Stretch (with towel)	Alternate 5X each way—right/left	5 sec. hold
	6 Two-Arm Hug/ Reverse Two-Arm Hug	Alternate exercise 2X each—front/back	20 sec. hold
	7 Groin Stretch	Alternate 2X each way—right/left	20 sec. hold
	8 Sprinter	2X one way—right, 2X other way—left	20 sec. hold
	9 Parallel Leg Stretch	2X one way—right, 2X other way—left	20 sec. hold
	10 Achilles' Tendon or Heel Cord Stretch	Alternate 2X each way—right/left	20 sec. hold
Sitting	11 Hamstring Stretch	2X one way—right, 2X other way—left; 2X together	20 sec. hold
	12 Hurdler/Reverse Hurdler	2X each way (right, left) 2X each way (right, left)	20 sec. hold
Lying on back	13 Back Stretch	Alternate 2X each way—right/left; 2X together	20 sec. hold

*Note: You may be able to stretch only 5 to 10 seconds in the beginning; if so, increase the repetitions accordingly (up to 4 or 5). However, your goal is to increase the length of the stretch, up to 30 seconds is good, and decrease the repetitions to 1 or 2.

WORKOUT CHART
JIM PALMER FLEXIBILITY FITNESS EXERCISES
F/AE (Flexibility/Aerobic Exercise)

POSITION	WORKOUT	BEGINNER	INTERMEDIATE	ADVANCED
Lying on back	1 Pelvic Tilt—5 sec. hold	5–10X	10X	10X
	2 Partial Sit-up—5 sec. hold	5–10X	10X	15X
	3 Full Sit-up	5X	10–15X	15–20X
	3A V Sit-up	—	—	5–10X
	4 Bent Knee-up	5–10X	10X	15X
	5 Bow & Arrow	5–10X	10–15X	15X
	5A Double-Leg Lowering	—	—	5–10X
	6 Rollover/Reverse Rollover	10/10X	15/15X	20/20X
	7 Barbell Arms	30X	40X	50X
	8 Paddle Arms—front/back	20/20X	30/30X	40/40X
	9 Punch Up Arms	30X	40X	50X
Lying on side	10 Side Leg Lift	20X	30X	40X
Sitting	11 Reverse Leg Lift	20X	30X	40X
Lying on abdomen	12 Back Leg Lift—Bent Knee	10–15X	15–20X	20–30X
	13 Back Leg Lift—Straight Knee	10–15X	15–20X	20–30X
	14 Back Lift—3 sec. hold	10X	15X	20X
	15 Push-up	5–10X	10–15X	15–25X
Standing	16 Arm Circle—Reverse Arm Circle	15/15X	20/20X	30/30X
	17 Juggle Arms	30X	40X	50X
	18 Windmill Arms	30X	40X	50X
	19 Side Bend	15X	20X	30X
	20 Double-Leg Half-Squat	15X	20–25X	30–40X
	21 Single-Leg Half-Squat	5–7X	8–10X	15X
	22 Heel Raise	15X	20–25X	25–30X
	23 Biceps Raise	10X	15–20X	25–40X

Complete workout with:
- 20 minute aerobic exercise
- Cooldown

NOTES:

#1–5A: If abdominal muscles get sore, move to another exercise and then return.

#7–9: Intermediate and advanced goals may be done with resistance, such as 2 lb. to 5 lb. household items (bag of flour). To begin, use light, manageable weights and lower the number of repetitions.

• #3A, 5A: For Advanced only.

#3: Vary arm positions.

#15: Vary hand positions.

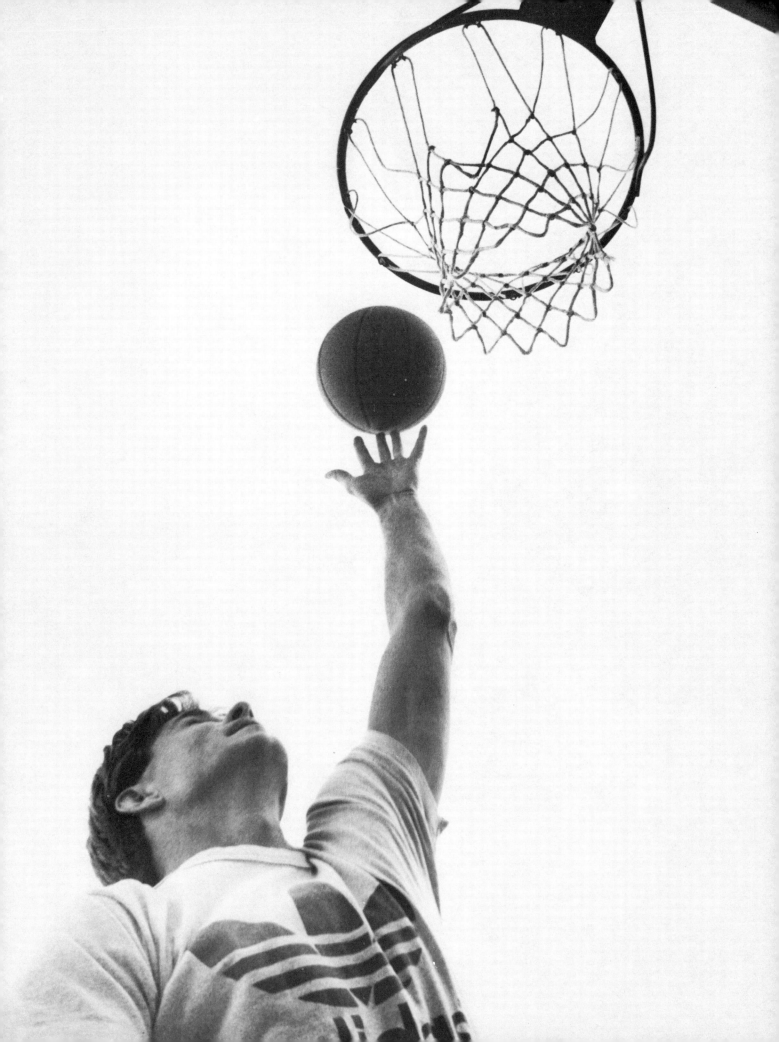

CHAPTER 3

PLAYING SPORTS TO STAY FIT...
BUT LET'S NOT GET HURT

Exercising is only one spoke in the wheel of fitness. All the benefits that accrue from exercising can be put to good use in playing sports or participating in recreational activities such as walking or hiking. It's a great way to stay fit, and the fun from competition and achievement really can motivate you to continue your exercise regimen.

I've heard too many people voice their regrets about not continuing their sports careers—and I'm not talking about professional athletes, but people like yourself who work in other fields to earn a living and feel that the only sports participation possible for them is to watch others play the games.

Nonsense! There is a lot of the little kid in all of us, and the fun we had playing sports as a youngster needn't become only a dim, pleasant memory. Of course, I have by choice played baseball most of my life, and to me it was great. There is nothing more pleasant than a warm, sunny afternoon at the ball park, and there was

nothing more exhilarating than competing, and with that came the camaraderie with teammates and our experiences together. If there is one thing I miss most about leaving the game as a player, it is spending time with people who were my friends and sharing those experiences.

But I resolved that when my professional sports career had ended, I would not walk away from sports as a participant, and I am urging you to feel the same way. Also, it is important that you prepare for that participation so that you will get more from it to benefit your overall physical being without fear of injury.

By preparation I mean strengthening the areas that will be put under stress while you are playing, and stretching the muscles you will use so that they will be elastic and ready for the sudden stops and starts that will occur during your activity. I have seen many people get upset when they go out to play and tear a calf or rib muscle or hurt their shoulder. Not only is that day ruined, but the injury can be serious enough to curtail their activities for two or three weeks or even longer.

What does this require?

How about 10 extra minutes before you begin playing? That's really all we're talking about—just enough time to stretch and strengthen the areas of your body which will be used most in your playing. Usually you find yourself waiting for 10 or 15 minutes before beginning, so I am going to give you some stretching and strengthening exercises that can easily be done during that time. The surest way is to give yourself the time for this necessary preparation, and the results, I believe, will enhance your performance and reduce your chance of injury.

The two most common causes of problems and/or injuries with sports activities come from not being prepared; that is, by having a weak muscle that is overworked and hasn't been strengthened, or by having a tight muscle that hasn't been stretched. I've never understood why people consider this necessary preparation time to be a burden, and I mean even current or former professional athletes who certainly should know better.

I've played racquetball with some who are content to show up, hang around until our court is available and then go out and do a bit of a warmup with the ball before beginning play. If you've ever played any of the racquet sports, you know that you put intense pressure on your legs, particularly your back and Achilles' tendons, with the sudden starts, stops and twists, and by not loosening that Achilles', for example, you are almost asking for trouble.

Dr. Arthur Pappas, Boston Red Sox team physician and one of the leading sports medicine practitioners in the nation, has always advised athletes—and he means pros as well as amateurs—that in order to play to the best of their ability and enjoy what they are doing to the utmost, they must prepare their bodies for the activity. I never pitched a game without going through my stretching routine, and I know many an athlete who will not even throw a ball—be it just to demonstrate the proper technique—without first unlimbering his arm as he would do if he were about to engage in a brisk workout or game. To

him, that arm is his livelihood and he will do nothing to jeopardize a meal ticket.

Your body also is part of your livelihood, and the fact that you are working to care for it will have a direct benefit when you engage in some form of athletic competition. Just take the process a few steps forward and prepare specifically for the activity in which you choose to participate.

Most parts of the body are actively involved in all sports, but to help you to prepare yourself, I have set up a program that identifies which exercises will be especially helpful in preventing injuries in your favorite sports.

The accompanying chart, *Injury-Free Sports Warmup Exercises: Stretching and Strengthening for Sports,* presents a Core Program, set in boldface capital letters, and a series of Additional Exercises which may be substituted or added to the Core Program for an alternate workout.

CORE EXERCISES: INJURY-FREE SPORTS WARMUP PROGRAM

I have listed 20 essential, or core, exercises for sports warmup. Numbers 1-8, 26-27, in bold face on the Sports Warmup Chart on page 39, are exercises whose descriptions can be found in Chapter 2. Descriptions of the remaining core exercises, Numbers 9-17 and 33, follow.

Standing Position

(9) *Ankle Circle:* Stand with feet at shoulder width; lift one foot with the toe just touching the ground; then push the ball of that foot into the ground and slowly rotate the foot and ankle clockwise. Reverse the action counter-clockwise and repeat with other foot.

(10) *Back Arm Reach, Palms Turned In:* Stand erect, feet at shoulder width, arms at your sides with palms facing your leg. Stretch your arms behind you.

(11) *Back Arm Reach, Palms Turned Out:* Feet and arms in same position, with hands rotated outward and palms away from your legs. Reach arms behind you.

(12) *Elbow Pull—Behind Head:* Stand erect, feet at shoulder width. Raise one hand as high as possible, grasping one end of a towel. Reach behind

SPORTS WARMUP CHART
INJURY-FREE SPORTS WARMUP EXERCISES:
STRETCHING AND STRENGTHENING FOR SPORTS

POSITION	EXERCISE	ESPECIALLY HELPFUL FOR:	
		SPORTS THAT REQUIRE MORE LOWER-BODY WORK	SPORTS THAT REQUIRE MORE UPPER-BODY WORK
Standing	1 Twister	*	*
	2 Side Bend	*	*
	3 Overhead Stretch		*
	4 Reverse Two-Arm Hug	*	*
	5 Groin Stretch	*	*
	6 Sprinter	*	*
	7 Parallel Leg Stretch	*	*
	8 Achilles' Tendon Heel Cord Stretch	*	*
	9 Ankle Circle—clockwise/ counter-clockwise	Alternate 5X each way	
	10 Back Arm Reach—Palms In		Alternate each way 20 sec. hold
	11 Back Arm Reach—Palms Out		Alternate each way 20 sec. hold
	12 Elbow Pull—Behind Head		Right, left 20 sec. hold
	13 Elbow Pull—Behind Back		Right, left 20 sec. hold
	14 Elbow-Wrist Stretch, Hand Up		Right, left 20 sec. hold
	15 Elbow-Wrist Stretch, Hand Down		Right, left 20 sec. hold
	16 Circular Arm Swing—clockwise/counter-clockwise		Alternate 5X each way
	17 Single-Arm Hug		Right, then left 20 sec. hold
	18 Double Squat	*	*
	19 Single Squat	*	*
	20 Toe Raise	*	
	21 Shoulder Roll—front Shoulder Roll—back		10X
	22 Sawing—front/back Sawing—side/side		10–15X
	23 Arm Crossover		15X
	24 Kneading		15–20X

*Exercise movements are described in Chapter 2.

POSITION	EXERCISE	ESPECIALLY HELPFUL FOR:	
		SPORTS THAT REQUIRE MORE LOWER-BODY WORK	SPORTS THAT REQUIRE MORE UPPER-BODY WORK
	25 Ball Roll		10–20X
Sitting	**26 Hamstring Stretch**		*
Lying on Back	**27 Back Stretch**	*	
	28 Pelvic Tilt—Sit-up		*
	29 Barbell Arms		*
	30 Punch Up Arms		*
	31 Paddle Arms		*
	32 Side Leg Lift	*	*
Lying on Side	**33 Side Hip Stretch**	**1X right, then left— 30 sec. hold**	
Lying on Abdomen	34 Back Leg Lift	*	*
	35 Back Lift		*
	36 Three-Hand-Position Push-up		15X 5 in each hand position
	37 Shoulder Blade Pinch No. 1		3X 10 sec. hold
	38 Shoulder Blade Pinch No. 2		3X 10 sec. hold
	39 Shoulder Blade Pinch No. 3		3X 10 sec. hold

*Exercise movements are described in Chapter 2.

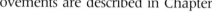

Ankle Circles

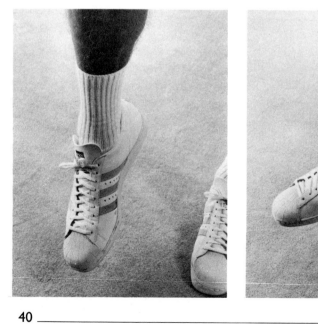
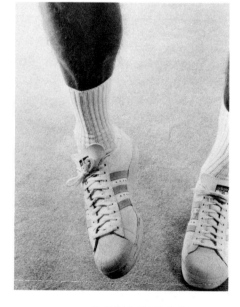

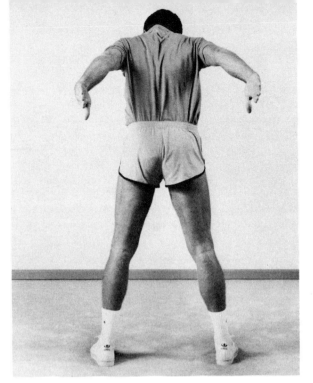

Back Arm Reach with Palms Turned In

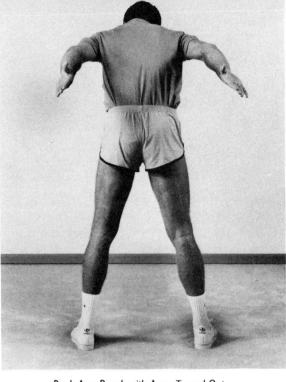

Back Arm Reach with Arms Turned Out

back with other hand and pull down on towel, keeping elbow pointing to ceiling. Alternate arms.

(13) *Elbow Pull—Behind Back:* Feet at shoulder width. Move one arm behind your body with elbow bent at 90 degrees. Move your other hand behind your back, grasping wrist, and attempt to pull arm toward middle, holding 20 seconds. Return arm to your side. Perform same movement with other arm.

Elbow Pull Behind Head

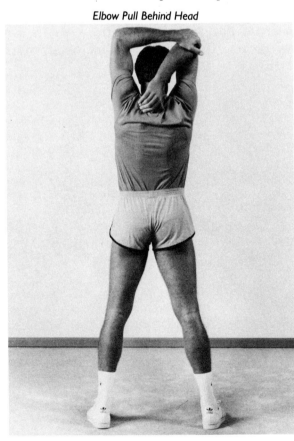

Elbow Pull Behind Back

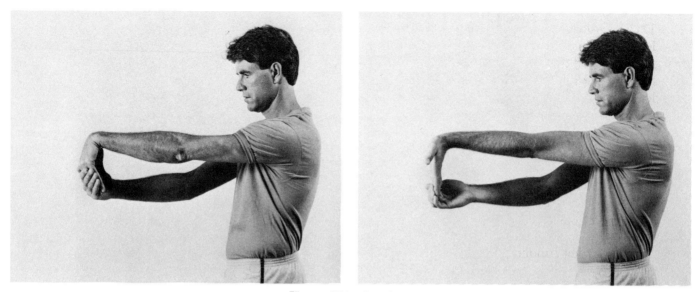

Elbow and Wrist Stretches

(14) *Elbow and Wrist Stretch, Hand Up:* Feet at shoulder width. Raise one arm in front of you at 90-degree angle with palm facing up. With other hand, gently stretch raised hand by pulling fingers backward. Hold 20 seconds, then lower arm.

(15) *Elbow and Wrist Stretch, Hand Down:* Start in with arms extended to front, palms facing down. Stretch the wrist by pointing the fingers toward the floor, grasping the back of the folded hand and pulling backward. Hold 20 seconds. Repeat with other arm.

(16) *Circular Arm Swing:* Feet at shoulder width. Lean over at the waist and let your arm hang down, swinging it in a counter-clockwise direction, then clockwise. Repeat with other arm. *Note:* The movement of the arms must come strictly from the shoulder.

Circular Arm Swing

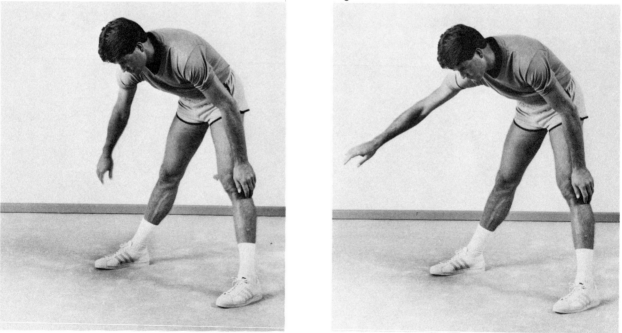

(17) *Single-Arm Hug:* Stand erect, feet at shoulder width, and lift your right arm 90 degrees in front of you. Move the arm across the front of your body so your hand is moving toward the left shoulder. Use left hand to grasp right arm just above the elbow, and stretch it at the shoulder joint in front of your body. Hold the pull 20 seconds, then put arm down. Repeat with opposite arm.

Lying on Side

(33) *Side Hip Stretch:* Lie on floor on left side, left hand in front, right hand resting across upper body. Bend right leg (underneath leg) approximately 90 degrees at knee; allow left leg to hang down over the right leg. Perform the same stretch on the opposite side.

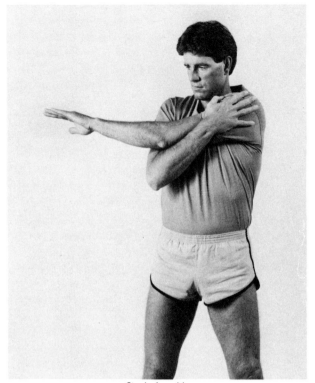

Single-Arm Hug

Side Hip Stretch

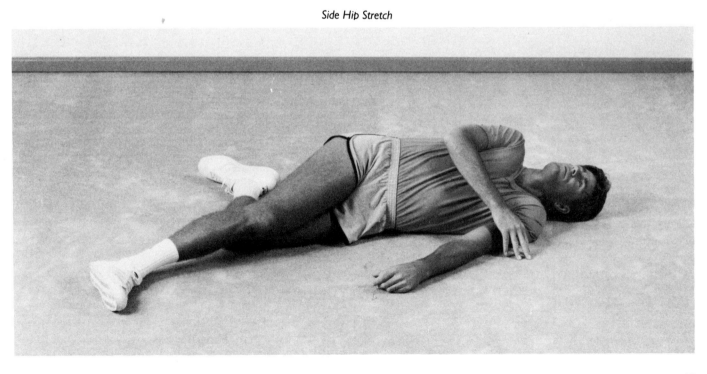

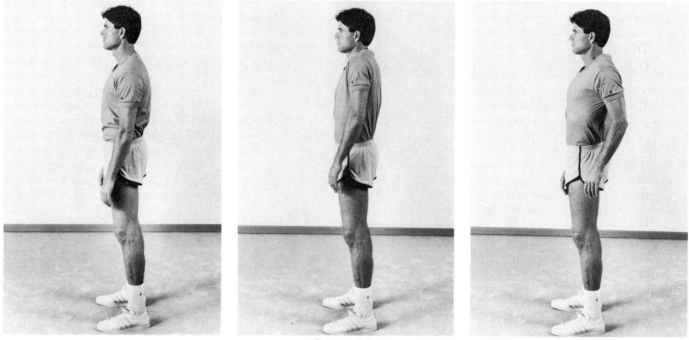

Shoulder Roll

Sawing, Front to Back

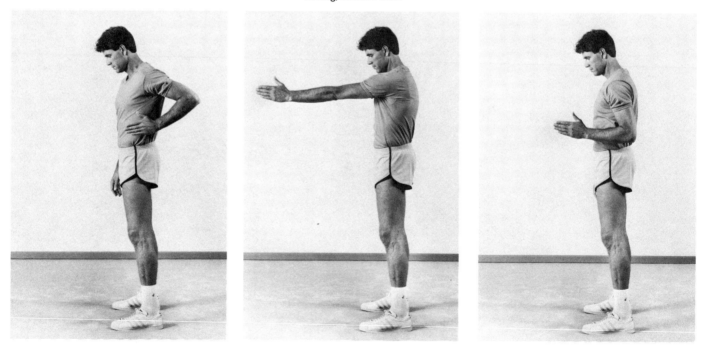

ADDITIONAL EXERCISES:
INJURY-FREE SPORTS WARMUP PROGRAM

Standing Position

(21) *Shoulder Roll:* Standing with legs at shoulder width and arms at your sides, lift one shoulder upward and rotate it backward; then repeat with the other shoulder. Do it alternating shoulders.

(22) *Sawing Front to Back:* Stand erect, feet at shoulder width and arms at sides, bent to 90 degrees at elbow. Move them forward and backward alternately from the shoulder, being certain to maintain the elbow flexed at 90 degrees. *Sawing Side to Side:* Hold your arm in front of your body with elbow bent to 90 degrees, and move arm from side to side, reaching each side of your body. Do each arm in each direction, being certain that the movement is occurring at the shoulder joint and not the elbow joint. Repeat with alternate arms.

(23) *Arm Crossover:* Stand erect, feet at shoulder width and arms extended 90 degrees to the side. Move both arms across the front of body as if to hug yourself, then return to starting position. Elbows will bend slightly as they come across the front of your body, but they should be straightened coming back to starting position.

(24) *Kneading:* Stand erect, arms extended in front of your body, slightly below waist. Flex arm and hand muscles and pull hands upward toward chest, clasping fist, and bend elbows as they move upward. At midchest, push them back toward floor, opening your fists and straightening fingers. Take 5 seconds to pull in upward direction and 5 seconds in downward move.

Sawing, Side to Side

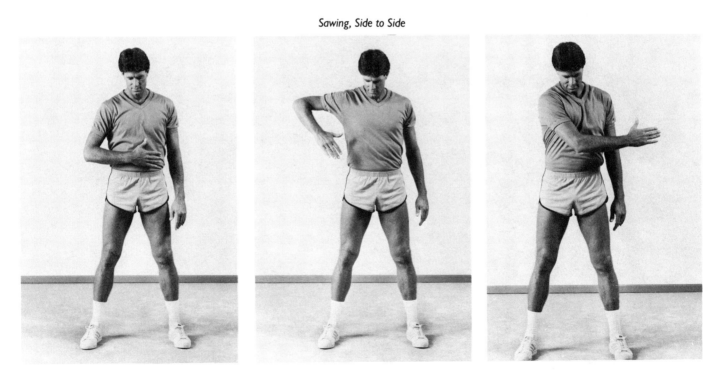

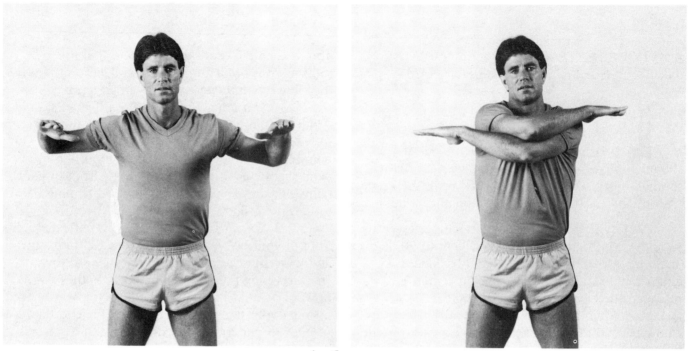

Arm Crossover

Arm Crossover

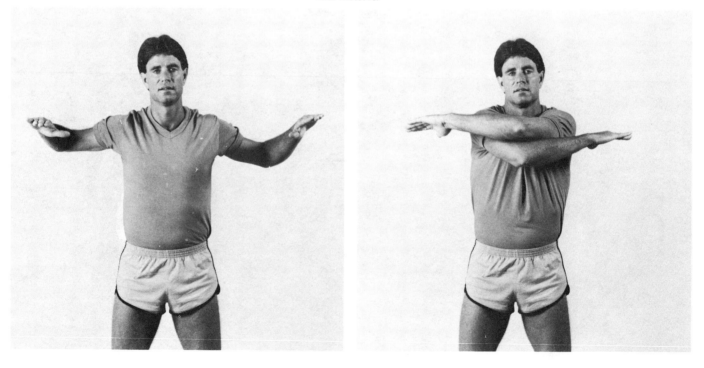

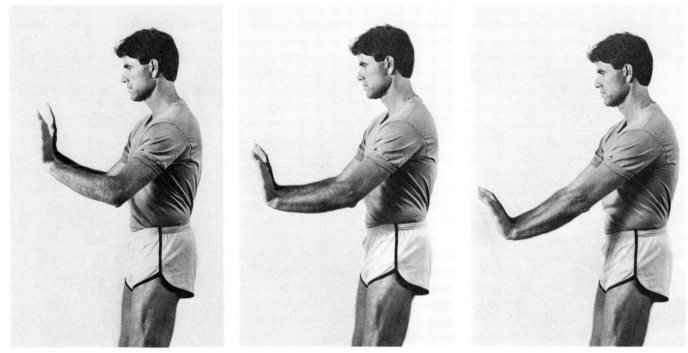

Kneading

Kneading

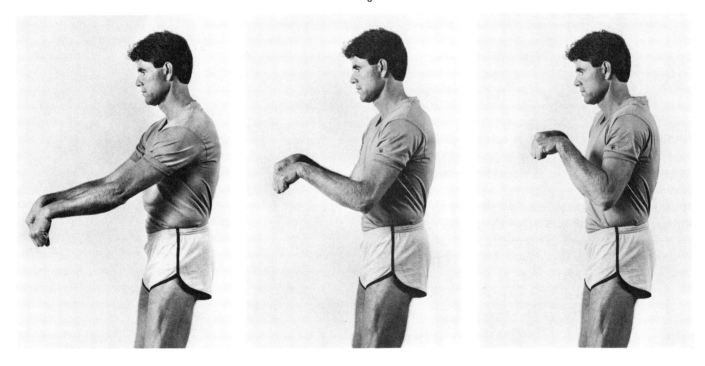

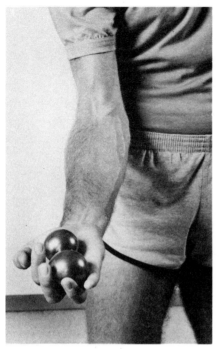

Ball Roll

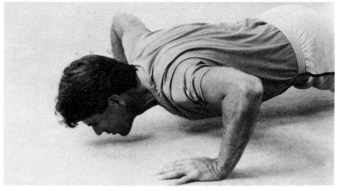

Push-ups/Hand Position 90°

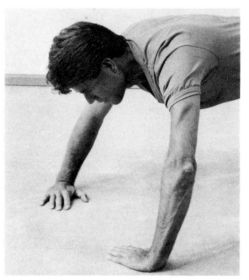

Push-ups/Hand Position 45°

Push-ups/Hand Position 180°

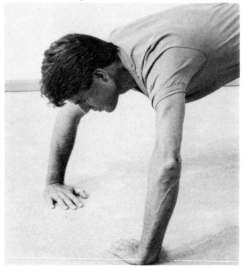

(25) *Ball Roll:* In standing position, and using 2 2-inch steel balls (golf balls can be substituted), place them in palm of one hand and rotate them around each other, using your fingers to cause motion. Do in each direction. Repeat with other hand.

Lying on Abdomen

(36) *Three-Hand-Position Push-up:* Face down, do this push-up as directed in the regular fitness section, but move the hands in three different positions during the repetition: first, as done in the fitness routine with fingers pointing straight ahead; second, with hands rotated 45 degrees inward; third, with hands rotated another 45 degrees so the fingertips are pointed toward each other. Change each hand position after 5 repetitions.

(37) *Shoulder-Blade Pinch No. 1:* Lying face down with arms out to side at 90-degree angle and elbows flexed at same angle, bring elbows, upper arms and forearms off the floor, pinching shoulder blades together. Hold for 10 seconds and bring arms back to the floor.

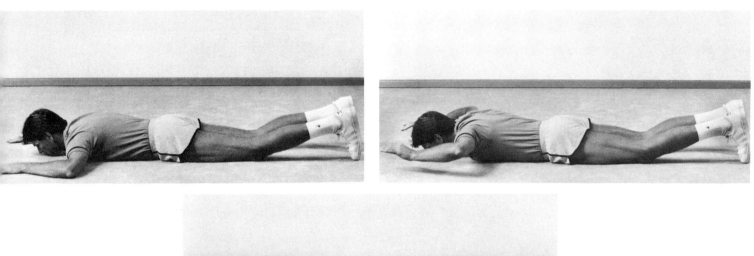

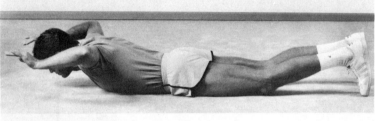

Shoulder-Blade Pinch No. 1

Shoulder-Blade Pinch No. 2

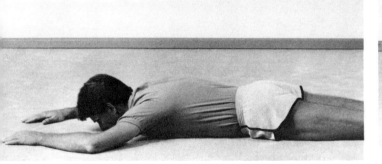

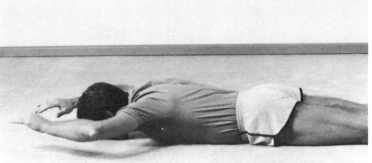

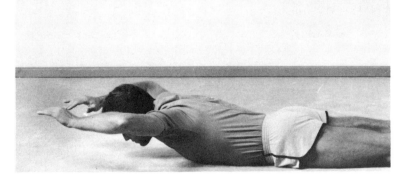

Shoulder-Blade Pinch No. 2

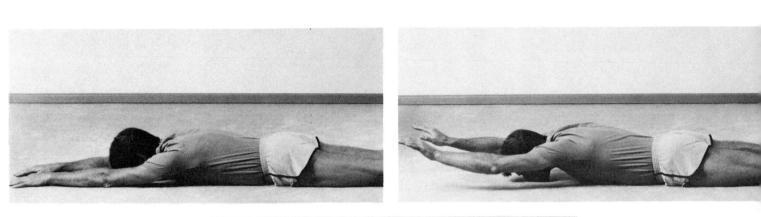

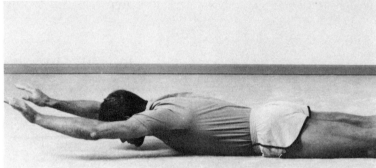

Shoulder-Blade Pinch No. 3

(38) *Shoulder-Blade Pinch No. 2:* Lying face down with arms and elbows in same position, raise arms above shoulder level about 45 degrees, lifting shoulders and arms off the floor, holding for 10 seconds.

(39) *Shoulder-Blade Pinch No. 3:* Lying face down on floor with arms in same position, stretch both arms upward so that upper arms nearly touch your ears. Lift arms and shoulders off floor and hold for 10 seconds.

One added starter: You may wish to increase your strength a bit by doing some simple weight work. If so, use a weight between 1 and 5 pounds, and increase the weight gradually. There is a law of diminishing returns in preparing for immediate sports participation using weights, so don't get caught up with any heavy-resistance exercises. They simply are not necessary for the activities which we have outlined.

And now that you have done something to help your game, go out and play ... and have a ball...or a racquet...or whatever makes you happy!

PLAYING

Like everyone, I have my own favorite list of sports, but it may be more extensive than yours, because I have had more time between baseball seasons to pursue these activities—activities, by the way, which were integral in keeping me in shape from season to season, and that was something I considered as a key part of my profession.

At any rate, at one time or another and with some measure of enjoyment, I have participated, as an adult, in walking, jogging, running, swimming, cycling, racquetball, bowling, golf, tennis, volleyball, soccer, softball (here I get a chance to hit because there is no designated hitter!), Frisbee and basketball. As a pro athlete whose legs were part of my livelihood, I have not taken to skiing, either cross-country or alpine, mainly because of the dangers that could have befallen my legs. My good friend Jim Lonborg almost ended his career— and did much to alter it—with an untimely skiing accident which required knee surgery in 1968,

only a few months after he had won the American League's Cy Young Award and helped pitch the Red Sox to the 1967 American League pennant. Ironically, he had invited me to join him on that western ski trip, but I had decided to go to Puerto Rico to play baseball.

I also don't play handball or squash, or hike, or ice- or roller-skate, or play flag or touch football.

To make it easier, I'm going to break down the sports which I play into three categories: On Your Own, One on One and Team.

On Your Own

Walking-running-jogging, swimming and cycling are the three in this category, and all should be preceded by the stretching and strengthening exercises for the lower body which we have just outlined.

Walking and jogging should precede *running* in your exercise progression, and both can be fun because they take you somewhere so you can get a look at the neighborhood, your community and the landscape. They also are terrific exercises as well as an aid to weight control and a boon to your cardiovascular system. Add a psychological lift as well, because joggers say they have a wonderful sense of well-being when they have finished.

It is generally accepted that a pace which covers a mile in 8 minutes or less is running, and anything that takes longer for a mile is jogging.

No one can tell you exactly how far you should run at the beginning. But you may find that you have to start out by walking. If that's the case, don't be discouraged. Very few beginners are able to run continuously for any distance.

You should probably begin with the "walk test." If you can comfortably walk 3 miles in 60 minutes, it's okay to start running. Or, more precisely, to start alternately jogging and walking. If you can't pass the test, simply walk 3 miles a day until you can.

In the beginning you should alternately run and walk continuously for 20 minutes. Speed isn't important, but the amount of time is. It takes about 20 minutes for your body to begin realizing the "training effects" of sustained, vigorous exercise.

So, after your warmup, walk briskly until you are moving easily. Then run at a comfortable pace until you begin to become winded and/or tired. Walk until you're ready to run again. Repeat the cycle until your 20 minutes are up. Take your pulse and check it against your Target Heart Rate (60 percent of Maximum Heart Rate) to ascertain whether you are deriving maximum aerobic training benefits.

The more often you run, the faster you will improve. At least 5 workouts a week are recommended for people who are trying to *raise* their level of fitness. For those trying to *maintain* their fitness level, 3 workouts a week are generally considered the minimum.

You should be able to talk while running or while alternately running and walking.

There's an easy way to find the right pace. It's called the "talk test." You should be able to talk while running or while alternately running and walking. If you're too breathless to talk, you're going too fast. As you progress, you'll find that you'll be able to carry on a conversation at higher and higher speeds.

That progress may seem slow at first, but in the weeks ahead you'll be amazed at how your strength and staying power increase. After 8 to 10 weeks, if you work out faithfully, you should be able to run the full 20 minutes at a reasonable pace, although this process may take somewhat longer for older persons or those not in good physical condition.

Once you've completed your reconditioning phase, you should extend your run to 30 minutes. Remember, the amount of time you spend is the key thing, not the time it takes you to cover a specific distance.

Running is something that comes naturally to most people. But it's important to be aware that there are different types of running. For example,

in most sports a person is taught to run for speed and power. But in running for fitness the objectives are different, and so is the form. Here are some suggestions to help you develop a comfortable, economical running style.

- Run in an upright position, avoiding excessive forward lean. Keep back as straight as you comfortably can and keep head up. Don't look at your feet.
- Carry arms slightly away from the body, with elbows bent so that forearms are roughly parallel to the ground. Occasionally shake and relax arms to prevent tightness in shoulders.
- Land on the heel of the foot and rock forward to drive off the ball of the foot. If this proves difficult, try a more flat-footed style. Running only on the balls of your feet will tire you quickly and make the legs sore.
- Keep your stride relatively short. Don't force your pace by reaching for extra distance.
- Breathe deeply with mouth open.

Where possible, run off paved surfaces and on grassy ones—a golf course, if there are no prohibitions, is ideal—because this places less strain on your legs, ankles, knees and lower back. Every time your foot hits the ground, it generates approximately 500 pounds per square inch of pressure, and a cushioned surface can make the impact easier to bear.

Also running off streets and roads is safer— you don't have to worry about traffic, nervous drivers, speeding trucks and, unfortunately, some crazy people who take delight in trying to bully runners off the road.

As for attire, in summer wear cotton—not nylon or synthetics because they will trap perspiration and interfere with your body's natural cooling system. In cold weather use the layered look— several layers of clothing to act as insulation and allow ventilation. These can include long-johns or thermal underwear, with a cotton turtleneck on top and cotton sweat pants on bottom.

If it's cold enough, wear a ski mask and gloves—but don't jog in very bitter cold when the wind chill or Fahrenheit is below zero. You can

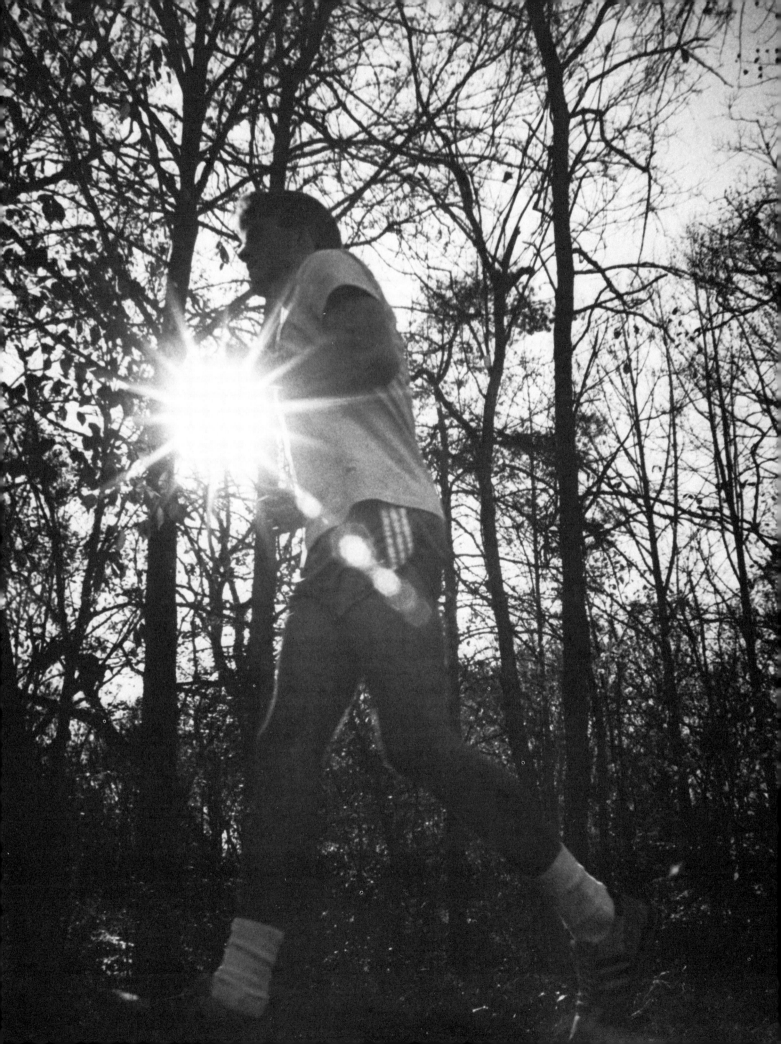

suffer frost burn to your respiratory system, as well as put your muscles under extreme jeopardy, regardless of your warmups.

One other caution before you start a jogging routine that you hope will lead to running: Get a medical checkup to reveal any hidden cardiovascular problems that may be hereditary. If you are thirty-five or older, it may be advisable to have medical tests, including a stress test, regardless of your conditioning state. And if there is a family history of heart disease, be sure to inform the doctor for a proper evaluation.

And on the good side, running does not cause heart disease. In fact, studies of groups of men in whom hereditary heart problems can be ruled out as a cause of heart disease show that running and aerobic exercise very definitely guard against heart disease.

Once you get your jogging routine down to a comfortable half-hour pace, you may wish to consider a faster running mode. Running, as noted previously, means covering a mile in 8 minutes or less. How do you build up to running longer distances?

The best way is to determine whether you have a "runner's build"—that is, whether you tend to be narrow rather than wide (not in a fat sense, just in your bone and muscle structure); have relatively thin wrists; and weigh about twice your height in inches. If all three are positive, then you have a "natural" runner's build, but only 10 to 15 percent of the population is said to fit that category, so don't feel left out if you don't, because the body adapts to regular exercise. You still can find success in running although your physique may differ from the above description.

Swimming, unlike jogging and running, must be learned before it can be mastered, so if you don't know how, join an adult class at your local YMCA, local recreation department or health club. Either way, many sports-medicine and aerobic experts say that the beginning swimmer, because of the extra effort expended in staying afloat and moving forward, receives greater benefit over the same time span than the expert who churns through the water with ease.

As with every sport and exercise, you must build up endurance and skill. Before beginning

your stretching and exercise warmups on the pool deck, walk back and forth in thigh-to-waist-deep water in the shallow end for several minutes to aid your aerobic activity, and then follow your swim with a 3-minute "cooldown" walk in the same way.

In building up endurance, set a specific distance goal, from 2 to 10 laps—and even more as you become more experienced. Swim at a comfortable speed until you tire; then continue with a slow breast stroke to recover; then resume swimming at original speed; slow again to the breast stroke...and so on, until you've reached your goal. If a breast stroke between "crawl" periods proves too strenuous, simply stop and tread water or walk in the shallow end of the pool until you're ready to move forward.

Cycling comes in two forms—stationary (indoors) and outdoor, and the latter can be recreational or competitive. The principles involved are the same for both, beginning with perhaps 10 minutes of pedaling at a moderate speed until you tire, then dropping to a slower speed until you've recovered. Alternate between the two until your time has expired. Stay at this level daily for as long as a week, then increase your time to about 13 minutes for several days, working up to 15 minutes. Eventually you'll go higher, but this is an exercise which you can do as much as 7 days per week.

Be comfortable when you ride, beginning with the proper attire. For serious fitness training: a pair of cycling shorts, seamless, covers the groin and upper thigh, and guards against chafing from the friction of the seat. And the seat—have a comfortable one, so extra cushioning may be necessary for some. There are wide-bodied seats especially made for indoor bikes, and there are soft-cushioned, larger sizes available for outdoor bikes.

When riding outdoors, some safety tips:

(1) Wear a helmet and, if you are beginning, long pants to stave off abrasions to the legs if you fall.

(2) Don't ride in the rain. Hand brakes are almost useless when wet.

(3) Stay off gravel or rutted surfaces as much as possible to avoid accidents.

(4) If you need to rest, hop off and walk your

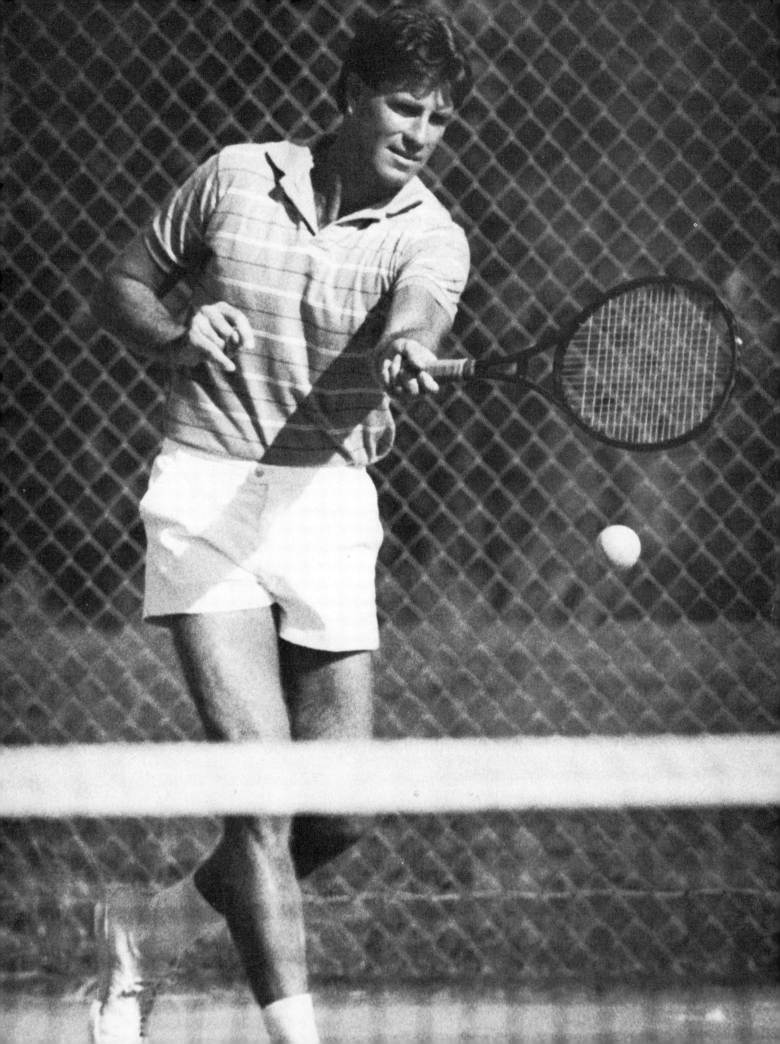

bike slowly, particularly if you are just starting out and must ride in a hilly area. If possible, start your training on flat surfaces and build up strength and endurance so you can keep moving up the hills.

One-on-One Sports

One of my favorites is *racquetball*. I play it as often as I can because it is terrific exercise and provides great competition. If you haven't tried it, find a friend who already knows how and who is willing to stay around while you gain some skill. When you do, you'll be in for a strenuous workout which not only helps to condition the heart and legs and burns calories at a high rate, but also is a lot of fun.

One must: Wear goggles because the ball, which comes at you at incredible speed, can fit perfectly into the human eyesocket. I need not be more graphic.

I have played *tennis* for years, but when I did so during my major-league seasons and at spring training, I used my left arm so as not to do anything ruinous to my pitching, or right, arm. Now I have no such worries, so I enjoy the sport in full swing.

Again, if you are a novice or wish to join the tennis craze, find a good instructor and practice regularly. Play with a partner who can return the ball to you so your skills will improve. Another method of achieving that—without a partner—is to hit balls off a wall or handball partition. Focus on returning the ball with a variety of shots. In effect, you have the perfect partner and never have to worry about line faults. Tennis is a good conditioning sport because when you become proficient you combine aerobic and anaerobic exercise. Nor does it have to be expensive, although the racquet is a necessary expense and, as I advised earlier in this chapter, you should get the best one that you can afford. If you are limited to playing in a city, check the wide variety of courts available and comparison-shop. In the country, check the outdoor courts at a high school or local beach, where there may be no cost; otherwise, comparison-shop for an inexpensive indoor court.

I am coupling *bowling and golf* because they are not high on the list of sports which condition, though I urge golfers to walk rather than ride a cart over the 18 or 27 holes to get as much exercise as possible. A golf course, not counting those forays into the woods and rough, measures approximately 3½ to 4 miles, and while it cannot be done at a brisk pace, walking it certainly has some benefit.

Occasional bowlers tell me that their legs feel the impact of this game because of the sudden stops while releasing the ball; and their lower arms also feel the strain of the 16-pound ball. Like golf, this sport, or game, involves skill and is not exceptionally taxing. But both are fun and serve as great outlets for the pressures and frustrations of the business week. That is worth something—provided you don't get even more upset when that little golf ball doesn't go exactly how and where you had hoped!

Team Sports

For conditioning, you can't depend on any one team sport to keep you in shape, though a steady diet of full-court basketball and goal-to-goal soccer won't do a bad job. However, for the camaraderie, team sports cannot be topped, and you can take that from someone who played one for more than half his life. For a person who works 40 or more hours a week at another job, getting together with friends and forming a team—with all that means in areas such as teamwork, succeeding together and striving to fulfill a common goal—offers great intrinsic benefits.

But if you worry more about conditioning yourself than other values, then *basketball* is a good team sport with which to begin. You must be in very good physical condition to play a full-court game over a long span of time. Pickup games don't stop as often as those in the schools and at professional levels; there is no referee to whistle fouls, so it is up and down, back and forth. I won't dwell on skills here, because the object of the game is not to set scoring records, but certainly you should have some proficiency in dribbling and passing, and be able to put up a fairly decent shot from near the basket.

A variation of this is half-court basketball, sometimes a necessity where playground space is limited. That is a stop-start game which begins when a team has the ball over the half-court line and puts it into play. Action slows under these conditions, but often players can go for longer periods without having to take a break.

Soccer is a terrific sport that promotes cardiovascular fitness and requires alertness, some speed and agility, and passing and dribbling skills. Size is not important, and any spacious lawn can serve as a field.

Neither *softball* nor *baseball* ranks high as a conditioning sport—it's what you do before the games which matters. But none is more fun to play, and they can be played forever. I'm not kidding, because last fall I was in St. Petersburg, Florida, to interview a softball team whose members were all over seventy-five years of age—and their catcher, George Barwell, was ninety-two! The men played in white shirts, bow ties and white trousers, and they did it in 90° weather. Further, they had a great time and no one had any physical problems.

Obviously, they have kept themselves in great physical shape and are active much of the year. Those men get more physical benefits from softball than you will, because neither it nor baseball gives you much more than some good anaerobic activity in running to catch a ball or trying to leg out a double or triple. Pitching and catching are the two positions where one gets more continual physical motion, but every position can be fun. If you haven't tried it, do so. You'll love it!

On the beach, where you also can surf and swim with good exercise results, *volleyball and Frisbee* are fine sources of exercise. Volleyball requires more continuous movement and Frisbee requires a great deal of hand-eye coordination plus some anaerobic activity as you move to catch the sometimes elusive disc.

Volleyball requires a great deal of jumping when you play at the net; and if you play on a beach where the sand is soft, your legs will get a good workout as you move to get to the ball. Socially, it is top-drawer, and all you really need are two poles, a net and a ball. Show up with the equipment, and the players will soon appear.

Popular Sports and How They Contribute to Total Fitness

Whether you're currently involved in a sport or simply trying to choose one, you may find the following information helpful in determining how a particular sport fits into the total fitness picture, and what benefits you may derive.

Each sport is rated in terms of how it contributes to the three components of physical fitness: (1) *Muscular Strength*, (2) *Cardiovascular Endurance (CE) or Aerobic Fitness* and (3) *Flexibility* (ability to achieve a full range of movement of the joint). For each of the three components, the sport is rated as Excellent, Good, Fair or Little Benefit (LB).

Naturally, these are broad ratings. A person may get more or less benefit depending upon how much energy he or she puts into the sport, and for how long. These sports are the most popular among Americans today, as compiled from the President's Sports Award program.

1. Backpacking and Climbing

Special note: In this sport the degree of benefit is partially determined by the terrain you cover (hills, mountains, flat areas, etc.) and by the weight of the pack. For maximum benefit the pack should weigh at least 10 percent of body weight.

a. Muscular Strength: Good, especially for legs and torso.
b. CE: Fair to Good.
c. Flexibility: Good, particularly when arms and upper body are used in climbing.

2. Basketball

a. Muscular Strength: Fair overall; Good for legs.
b. CE: Good; stop-and-start nature of sport does not usually require sustained running for any length of time; Natural flow and action of game similar to internal training.
c. Flexibility: Excellent; jumping, shooting, blocking require flexibility in arms, legs, entire body.

3. Bicycling

a. Muscular Strength: Good; mainly for legs; arms benefit, too, but not nearly as much.
b. CE: Excellent; even with gears, vigorous bicycling (not coasting) makes healthy demand on heart and CV system.

c. Flexibility: Fair; legs get most of the benefit since arms and upper body are mostly stationary.

4. Bowling

a. Muscular Strength: LB; arms, back and legs get some benefit, but not much.
b. CE: LB; no sustained demand on CV system.
c. Flexibility: Fair.

5. Canoe-Kayak-Rowing

a. Muscular Strength: Excellent in arms and torso—especially if paddling upstream or against a current; can be excellent for legs and lower body in rowing, if legs are also used to push off on each stroke.
b. CE: Excellent when done for extended period of time, against current, or in a race.
c. Flexibility: Excellent for upper body; lower body, too, if legs are used.

6. Golf

a. Muscular Strength: Fair; for arms, shoulders, and torso when swinging; otherwise, there is little benefit (LB).
b. CE: Fair, but only if you walk around the course; benefit increased somewhat if you carry your own clubs.
c. Flexibility: Good.

7. Gymnastics

a. Muscular Strength: Excellent; almost all gymnastics activities require strength in arms, legs and rest of body.
b. CE: Good; degree of benefit naturally depends upon length of time spent actually performing an activity, but most tumbling routines and routines on apparatus are long enough to make necessary demands on cardiovascular system.
c. Flexibility: Excellent for entire body.

8. Handball-Racquetball-Squash

a. Muscular Strength: Good; stop-start movements required by each sport make sudden demands on muscles of entire body, especially legs.
b. CE: Excellent when played vigorously for up to an hour.
c. Flexibility: Good for entire body.

9. Jogging and Running

a. Muscular Strength: Fair; good for legs and helps arms and upper body somewhat.
b. CE: Excellent; one of the best cardiorespiratory activities a person can pursue.
c. Flexibility: Fair.

10. Martial Arts (Judo, Karate, etc.)

a. Muscular Strength: Fair; strength is often not the main focus of martial arts, but it is important and most martial arts help develop it to some degree.
b. CE: LB; even in competition, most martial arts do not demand aerobic endurance over a sustained period of time.
c. Flexibility: Excellent; most require good flexibility all over the body, and some even include flexibility exercises before participation begins.

11. Rugby

a. Muscular Strength: Good; most benefit comes from exercises done to train for play.
b. CE: Excellent; a lot of intermittent running required.
c. Flexibility: Good.

12. Scuba and Skin Diving

a. Muscular Strength: Fair; must have some strength in legs and arms, but strength not a major requirement of the sport.
b. CE: Fair; certainly helpful, but sports do not require sustained aerobic activity.
c. Flexibility: Excellent; as with plain swimming, entire body is involved.

13. Skiing (Alpine and Nordic)

a. Muscular Strength: Excellent; muscles all over

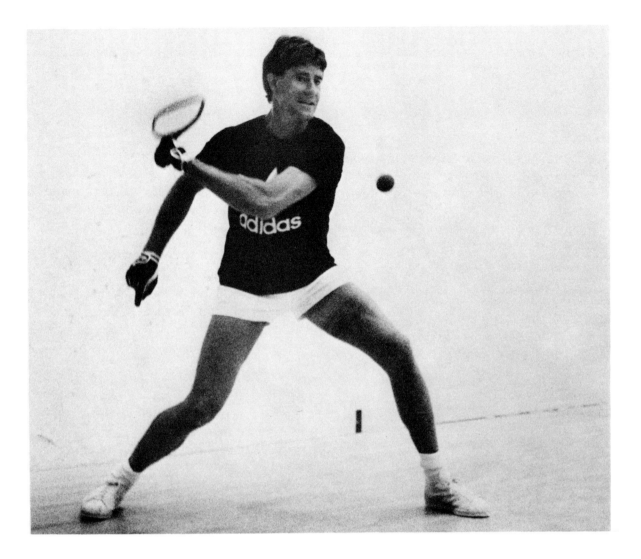

body are brought into play, especially those in the legs.

b. CE: Excellent, particularly in Nordic (cross-country) skiing.

c. Flexibility: Excellent; sports call for total body flexibility.

14. Soccer

a. Muscular Strength: Good; develops powerful legs, arms and upper body.

b. CE: Excellent; a lot of sprinting and continuous running required.

c. Flexibility: Excellent; sport requires coordination and flexibility of all parts of body.

15. Skating (Ice, Roller and Figure)

a. Muscular Strength: Good for legs, of course, but also for arms used for speed and balance, and for torso.

b. CE: Excellent, particularly when skating for speed.

c. Flexibility: Excellent, particularly in figure skating, where entire body must be carefully directed and controlled.

16. Softball

a. Muscular Strength: LB; some strength required to hit and throw, but generally not a strength-building sport.

b. CE: LB; even in base running, demand on cardiovascular system is not sustained long enough to do much good.

c. Flexibility: Fair to Good.

17. Swimming

a. Muscular Strength: Good; exercises muscles all over the body; strength especially important when swimming distance of ¾ mile or more.

b. CE: Excellent.

c. Flexibility: Excellent; requires good flexibility in arms, legs, entire body.

18. Table Tennis

a. Muscular Strength: LB.

b. CE: LB, unless played especially vigorously.

c. Flexibility: Fair for arms and upper body; lower body, too, if played vigorously.

19. Tennis

a. Muscular Strength: Fair to Good; legs derive strength benefits.

b. CE: Fair; in most cases, sustained cardiovascular exercise is not required.

c. Flexibility: Good; entire body must be flexible to play well.

20. Volleyball

a. Muscular Strength: Fair to Good; strength required in legs to jump and arms to hit, but control is often more important.

b. CE: Fair to Good; stop-start nature of the game inhibits a total aerobic workout.

c. Flexibility: Excellent; jumping, hitting, dashing to make a play—all require good flexibility.

21. Walking

a. Muscular Strength: Fair to Good; benefits legs, but not a strength-building activity for rest of body.

b. CE: Fair, up to 4 m.p.h. (15 minutes per mile) or less.

c. Flexibility: Good for entire body; be sure to allow arms to swing freely and naturally.

22. Water Skiing

a. Muscular Strength: Good; legs, arms, torso are all involved.

b. CE: LB.

c. Flexibility: Good; flexibility needed to get up on skis and to execute any tricks or maneuvers.

23. Weight Training

a. Muscular Strength: Excellent; of course, training should involve entire body.

b. CE: Fair to Good (see a qualified Nautilus or Universal Gym instructor).

c. Flexibility: Good to Excellent.

RESISTANCE AND STRENGTH TRAINING

As you probably have gathered, I am an enthusiastic exponent of my fitness program, which combines isotonics and aerobic exercise, plus sports participation as complementary units in a well-rounded approach. However, adding a resistance program, through weight training, will provide additional benefits for your body.

Suffice it to say I have mixed feelings about heavy-weight lifting, and that is a personal prejudice based on what I think is best for me, what I wish to achieve from conditioning, and how I have modeled my own routine. But I certainly bow to those who wish to pursue resistance training. I advise that they follow all prescribed cautions and that they understand the object of their performance with weights.

Don't get me wrong. I do not ignore all weight programs. Indeed, I still carry on some conditioning in a Nautilus center, something that I began years ago when I was at the peak of my pitching career with the Orioles, so I am familiar with all that is involved. Here, though, I'm going to give you some idea of how far you may wish to go in pursuing such conditioning; I am not going to develop or suggest any programs. Those you must get from a qualified instructor after you lay

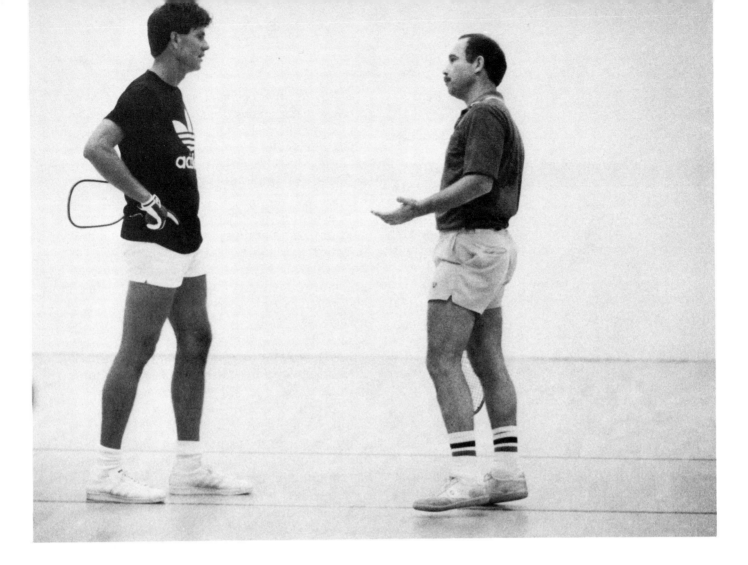

out your own goals. If you are thirty-five or over, or have a history of heart disease or diabetes, then first you must be cleared for such a program.

From a personal standpoint, I pursued my Nautilus regimen because it helped to give me a bit more strength in areas where I needed it, yet I did it at a pace that would allow me to maintain a fluid delivery in my pitches.

Such programs have highs and lows with athletes. Linemen and linebackers in football pursue them with great vigor because they wish to build up strength and bulk; they need both to move players out of their way. Quarterbacks are like pitchers in baseball. Their priority is to maintain flexibility as well as strength, yet they do not want their upper body tightened so they cannot deliver the ball.

When Kirk Gibson, the Detroit Tigers' fine outfielder, decided to play major-league baseball

after being drafted by the NFL, thanks to a fine football career at Michigan State, he found that the weight training he had done in that sport impeded his bat swing and was hurting his baseball career. So he went through a training program that in essence stretched his muscles and loosened his upper body.

Dr. Pappas, the Red Sox team physician, discourages all pitchers from doing heavy arm and shoulder weight lifting, and recommends light weights with more repetitions and the development of a total balanced shoulder function. What occurs otherwise, he has told me, is that pitchers who try to strengthen their shoulders with heavy weights wind up with greater strength in the front of their shoulder and a relative weakness in the back of the shoulder.

He also is wary of the competitiveness of athletes—it can lead them to take the weight programs too far and thus do more harm than good.

Decide what you want from your program.

I think you can see from this that you must decide what you want from your program, and how it will affect the kind of body which you wish to produce.

If you decide to pursue a serious weight-training program, here are some of the factors you should consider:

(1) *Decide your ultimate goals.* Remember, working on machines which strengthen your legs to increase speed will do nothing for upper-body strength; and working on your upper body will not increase your speed. Be certain that whatever program you choose will give you exactly what you want.

(2) *Read as much as you can* about weight training to learn about the best kind of equipment and the different techniques, particularly those most recently developed. You can use this information when you begin shopping around for the proper fitness center and a competent instructor.

(3) Visit a number of facilities—*comparison-shop*—to see what kind of equipment they have; how it is kept up; how crowded the place is at the time of day when you can best pursue this program. Be wary of shiny new equipment not sprayed with a lubricant, because equipment that sticks simply impedes the exercises. The same is true with off-center or damaged gear; and be especially leery of equipment that lights up when you complete certain programs. Gimmickry like that may be hiding an inferior product.

(4) *Check out the instructors* at these facilities. Lots of improperly trained personnel have been hired to staff the centers so as to keep business brisk. Ask to see their credentials and know their background, and if you have a question, check it out. Beware of anyone who promises instant results or says there is only one way to do something, regardless of the exercise area. Only you can provide yourself with the body you want, and only you know what you want accomplished.

(5) *Insist on maintaining a specific and overall program.* That means doing your cardiovascular program at least three times a week. If you want to build your body, don't neglect your legs in favor of the upper body; or if you want to become a stronger tennis player, don't neglect the left side of your body because you are right-handed. Agility and dexterity help everyone, whether or not you are an athlete. And mix some of those athletic exercises into your program. It will give it a fun flavor.

(6) *Wear proper clothing,* meaning loose-fitting and non-restricting items such as sweat pants, shorts and a T-shirt. Be sure to have good shoes, particularly if you will be doing a lot of work on your feet.

(7) *Don't do your work on an empty stomach.* Eat several hours before starting—4 is a good number—in order to get something to burn as energy.

(8) Be sure your *environment* for exercise is warm, yet properly ventilated. A cold gym means you take longer to warm up and you must be more careful about cooling down. That is all a part of selecting the proper facility.

(9) *Don't overstretch* while you are warming up. If you feel pain or the muscle trembles, back off. If you try to short-cut this, you'll be asking for trouble.

(10) Don't allow yourself to become *dehydrated* because that can impair your performance and lead to injury, illness or cramping. The temperature, the humidity and the type of clothing you wear will all affect the amount of liquid loss from your system. Water and fruit juices are best to replenish lost liquid, and be wary of commercial products which promote thirst reduction and increased energy. Some of those are nothing more than a mix of sugar and water.

(11) When *bending,* do it from the knees, not from the waist. Keep your back straight, and this is essential in weight training (as well as most other physical activity, as we shall see in our chapter on posture and body mechanics). Lifting even a 10-pound weight improperly could result in an injury. Be sure to maintain a supporting leg or arm under your body when it is leaning.

(12) *Don't overtrain,* and don't do more than you are able, or is suggested. That was the point I was making about Dr. Pappas' fear that athletes can become too competitive when working on these

programs and try too much. It is better to lift too little weight than too much. If you push yourself beyond the proper limits, you may be too hurt or too fatigued to finish the workout. Listen to your body and if your muscles become fatigued or start to burn, stop and turn to something else. Strength and endurance can vary day by day, even hour to hour, so don't think you are failing. Doing a little less one time may help rather than hurt and may even be your "maximum" for that one time.

(13) Be sure you get *proper rest.* Your needs may increase or decrease with exercise, and your body will tell you. Don't work through an injury; work around it if you must. But remember, the fact you aren't working a specific muscle doesn't mean that it is lying dormant. Rest is often the best medicine for an injury.

4-WEEK FITNESS WORKOUT CYCLE

The 4-week cycle chart illustrates how to integrate the basic Jim Palmer exercise and aerobic workout programs with participation in your favorite sports and aerobic activities, such as jogging, running, cycling, swimming, cross-country skiing and walking.

The Basic Fit program will give you a minimum level of fitness and prepare you for a more vigorous or stepped-up program. Adoption of the Extra Fit and/or Palmerfit schedules is a total commitment to improving your health and fitness.

4-WEEK FITNESS WORKOUT CYCLE

	SUN	MON	TUES	WED	THU	FRI	SAT
BASIC FIT	F/AE		F/AE		F/AE		
EXTRA FIT		F/AE		F/AE	S/AA	F/AE	S/AA
PALMERFIT		F/AE	S/AA	F/AE	S/AA	F/AE	S/AA
BASIC FIT		F/AE		F/AE		F/AE	
EXTRA FIT	F/AE		F/AE	S/AA	F/AE		F/AE
PALMERFIT	F/AE		F/AE	S/AA	F/AE	S/AA	F/AE
BASIC FIT		F/AE		F/AE		F/AE	S/AA
EXTRA FIT	S/AA	F/AE	S/AA	F/AE		F/AE	S/AA
PALMERFIT	S/AA	F/AE		F/AE	S/AA	F/AE	S/AA
BASIC FIT		F/AE	S/AA	F/AE	S/AA	F/AE	
EXTRA FIT	F/AE		F/AE	S/AA	F/AE		F/AE
PALMERFIT	F/AE	S/AA	F/AE		F/AE	F/AE	F/AE

KEY: F/AE = FLEXIBILITY/AEROBIC EXERCISE PROGRAM
     S/AA = SPORTS OR AEROBIC ACTIVITY

BASIC FIT: 12–15 TIMES PER 4-WEEK CYCLE
EXTRA FIT: 16–21 TIMES PER 4-WEEK CYCLE
PALMERFIT: 22–24 TIMES PER 4-WEEK CYCLE

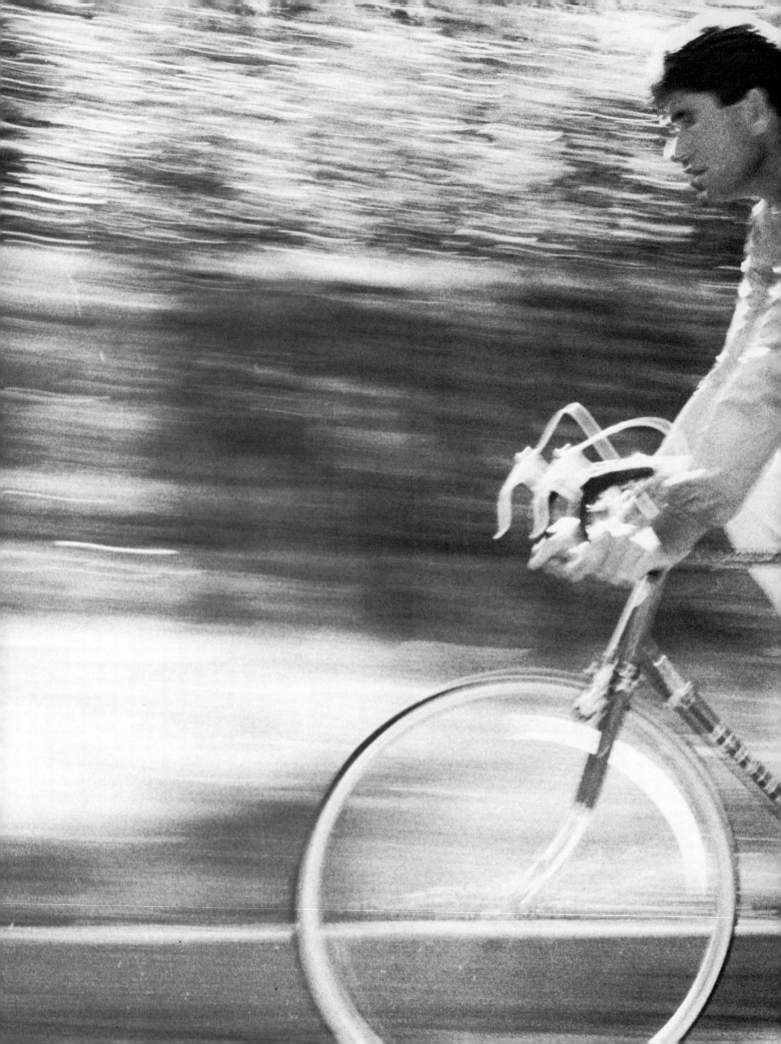

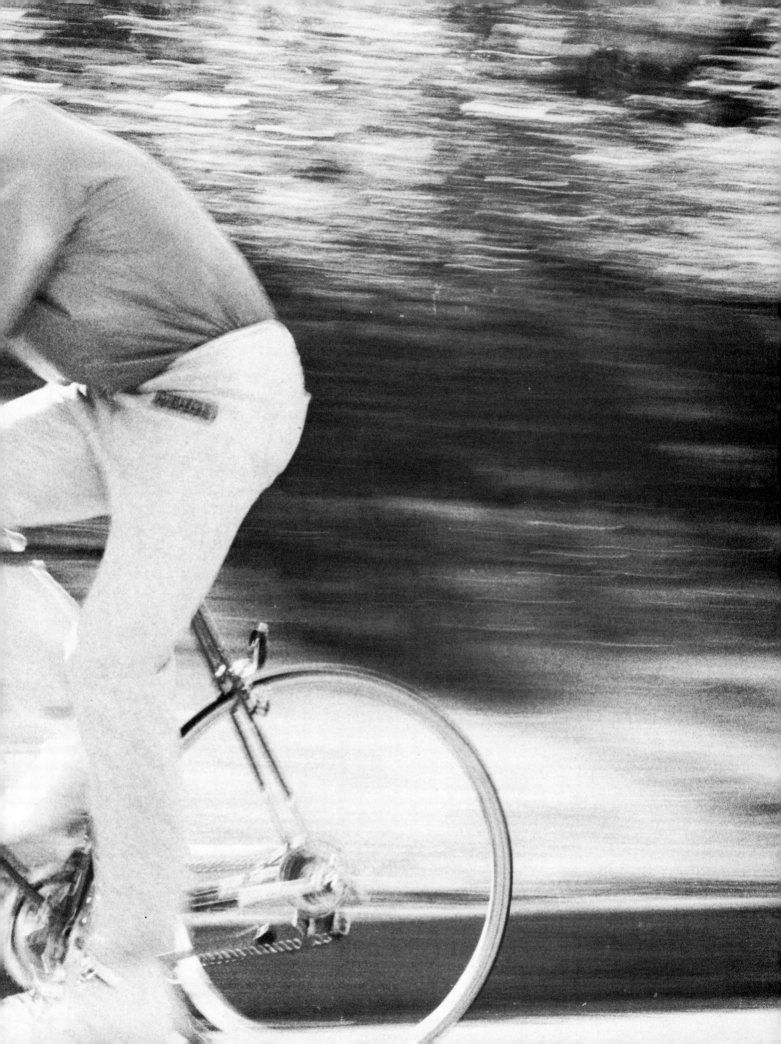

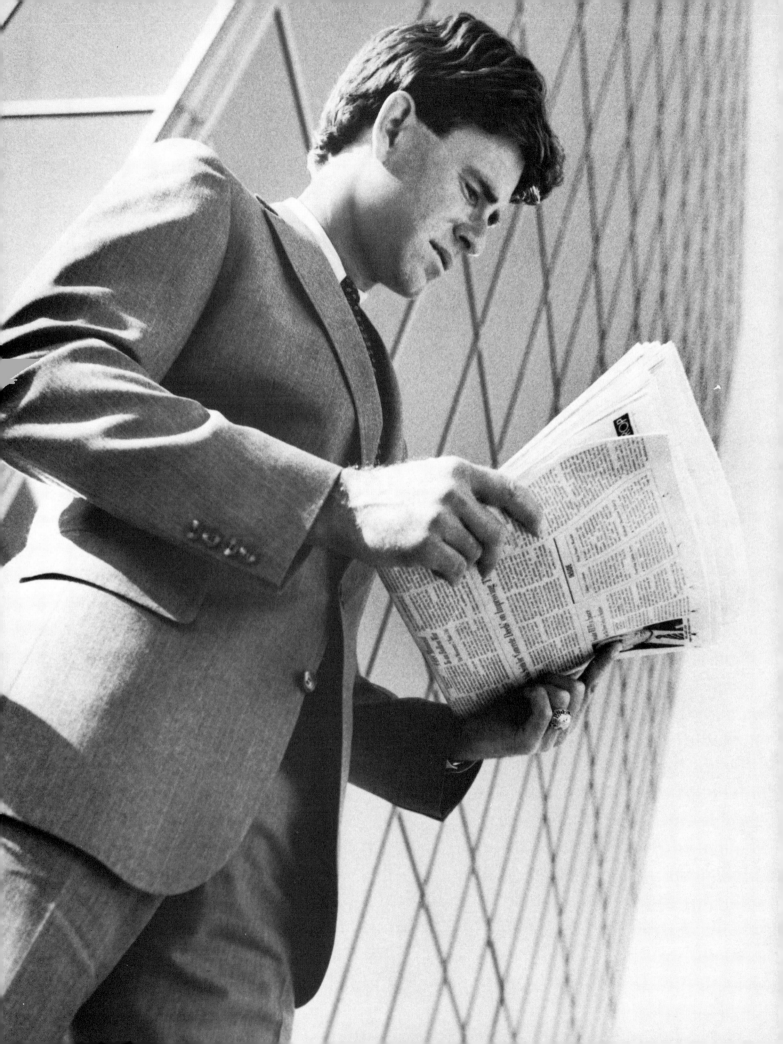

CHAPTER 4

BODY BALANCE AND POSTURE: STAND STRAIGHT, WALK TALL

"Stand up straight or you'll have bad posture!"

How many times did you hear that when you were growing up?

Nothing has changed, because I feel very strongly about the subject—and so should you— particularly since we have talked so much about improving your body's appearance. It doesn't make much sense to get into a conditioning program, perhaps add some resistance work to help polish your overall look, and then have the whole effect spoiled by poor body balance.

I guess I'm a bit sensitive about the subject because friends have told me I should do more. I'm 6'4"; I hunched over a pitching mound for nineteen years, taking signs from a catcher; and if I'm not careful, there are times when I walk around looking as if I'm still trying to get a sign.

Now that I'm no longer pitching and am into career work that carries me frequently into the public eye, I have become very aware of my carriage, and I can tell you that it does make a difference. I also have become very aware of how other people carry themselves and sit, stand and walk. I've gotten to the point where I can often tell a lot about someone who has good posture. That person seems to have a healthy outlook on life, and radiates a very positive demeanor, without a trace of self-consciousness about his carriage. When I see someone whose body balance is faulty, invariably, it seems, that person is rather apologetic about himself and walks with almost a shuffle as if to hide the poor posture, perhaps because of a sensitivity about his height, or from a lifetime of not paying attention to that body imbalance.

I'm also aware of posture and body-balance problems because I've had more than my share during my career, with injuries to my neck, back, hips and knees, as well as trying to stave off the miseries that can plague a pitcher, such as waking up with a sore pitching arm after a night's sleep or coping with a hotel's sub-rate pillows which can give you a sore neck. I know people wonder why pitchers are so sensitive to every twinge and tweak, but a pitcher's body is his livelihood, and when there is cash on the line, you learn to pay attention.

I wanted to know more, and what I learned was that good posture is really a matter of good alignment and the proper balance of muscles around the pelvis. And what constitutes "good alignment"?

Let's start from the top.

The *head* should be held in an erect position so the chin is parallel to the floor. Your *arms* should hang relaxed at the sides of the body with palms facing inward; *elbows* are slightly bent and *shoulders* level, neither forward or backward. The *chest* should be slightly up and forward with your *abdomen* held flat. The *back* is held fairly erect, both in the upper and lower regions so the spine holds its natural curves, in which the neck and upper back show a forward curve and the lower back and tailbone are curved backward.

Your pelvis should be equally balanced on the right and left, meaning the hips are level.

Your *pelvis* should be equally balanced on the right and left, meaning the *hips* are level; your body's weight should be borne equally on both *legs*, which should run straight up and down, with the *knees* forward. Your *feet* should toe out only slightly, with the weight evenly distributed.

How do you know whether this is you? Stand before a full-length mirror, with your back to the wall, and take first a front and then a side look.

If you don't have a full-length mirror handy—or even if you do—bad posture can show up in the form of an S-shaped spine, round shoulders and tilted hips. If you work in an office and are in the habit of talking on the phone while pressing it between your ear and shoulder, that can lead to a raised shoulder, as well as a stiff neck at day's end. Hold the phone in your hand and sit in

your chair—everywhere—with the hips well back, shoulders square and feet flat on the floor.

Your occupation can be a deterrent to good posture—anything that hunches your shoulders over a desk, table or drawing board, for instance, and no one is immune, including those who do the sewing, ironing and dishwashing. If that is you, drop your hands to your sides and roll your shoulders up, back and down, and do it fifteen or twenty times, twice a day. That will keep your shoulder and chest muscles limber and help to reduce the muscle tension in the upper back.

I know that a woman who carries a young child around can suffer posture problems from the weight of the child pulling down on the body. I was filming a television commercial for Maryland's Air National Guard several years ago and spent five hours on a day that went from cloudy and overcast to clear and cold with wind gusts of about thirty miles per hour. The filming was done in an unheated hanger and I carried a sixty-pound parachute on my left shoulder during the entire session. On the way home I stopped for my Nautilus workout and while I was doing my reps on one of the neck machines, something popped in my neck, opposite the side of my body where I had carried the parachute. I had very limited range in that region for nearly a month because I had compensated for the weight pulling down on one side of my body by resisting with the other side.

That form of muscular imbalance can take other guises and is the main physiological reason for poor posture, and there are other signs as well. One of the most obvious regarding poor foot posture is pronation of the feet, where they point outward and turn downward on the inner edges. This lessens a person's power in his stride and can cause pain in the ankle and the inside of the lower leg, and also flat feet. To correct the condition, try picking up marbles with your toes; or walk barefoot on the outer edges of your feet, with your toes pointed forward.

We really want to focus on specific areas—the head, the trunk, and the shoulder and pelvic girdles, the most important segments to have in good muscular and mechanical balance because they are the foundation on which force is directed to the arms and legs. Without bogging you down

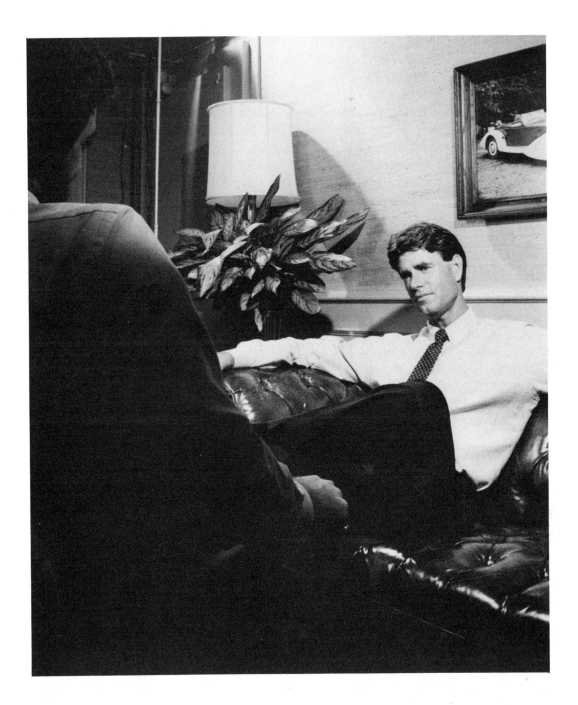

in a physiological and anatomical discussion, there are two groups of muscles in the front of your body, the abdominal and the hip flexors, which serve to balance two other sets at the back of the body, the hamstrings and the back extensor. Together they are known as the *pelvic force couple.*

These opposite groups of muscles work to tilt the pelvis forward or backward, and any disturbance in any of them can misalign your posture.

For instance, if the back extensors (muscles in lower back) and hip flexor muscles (in front and top of thighs) are much stronger, then the abdominal and hip extensor muscles often are weak, causing the pelvis to push forward; and if the situation is reversed in muscle strength, then the pelvis pushes backward, very often called a "flat back."

Something like round shoulders is brought

about by tightness in the chest; a tightness in the chest muscles and a weakness in the back muscles will cause a "forward head," and this causes a tightness in the back of the neck.

Before continuing any further, if you feel any undue pain or postural deviation, get your answers from a physician or physical therapist. They are professionals equipped to evaluate your body balance and posture and recommend the correct remedial action.

FIGURING YOUR POSTURE

Stand with your back against the wall in your natural position, feet flat on the floor, without shoes, about 2 inches from the wall. If your head is not touching the wall, you may have a slightly forward head with muscle tightness in the back of your neck. You should stretch these muscles with a *chin tuck* exercise, in which you pull your head up as if there were a string attached to the top rear portion, and tuck your chin down against your neck.

If your shoulders are not touching the back of the wall, they are probably forward and rounded, meaning that the muscles in the front of your chest and those around the front of your shoulder joint probably are tight. To help correct this, do the *Reverse Hug* and *Overhead Stretch* exercises. To strengthen the stretched and weakened muscles of the upper back, do the *Back Arm Reach* with your palm facing out, plus the *Shoulder-Blade Pinch*. All of these have been detailed in previous chapters.

Now for the *lower back*—and here I can speak volumes from personal experience, most of which led me to seek information about posture and body balance.

I found out about my own postural problems early in my major-league career when, after an examination, it was discovered that one leg was a bit shorter than the other. My hamstrings were tight and the stress was reflected in my lower back with a constant pain, which I aggravated by slipping off a wet pitching mound. An orthopedist suggested that I just stuff a big towel behind my lower back whenever I drove my car—like the lumbar supports now featured in many new cars—and that helped to relieve a lot of the pain.

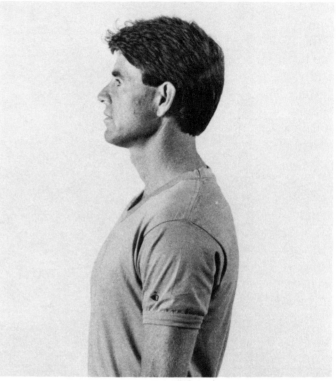

Chin Tuck

Chin Tuck

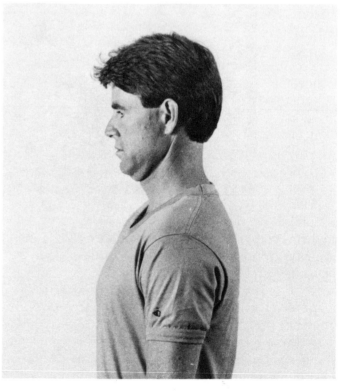

In 1979 I was playing racquetball with Marty Domres, a former NFL quarterback, and in our fifth game, when I was a little tired, I reached for the ball and felt something pinch in my back. I had moved an extra vertebrae—called a "floating vertebrae"—with which I was born, and nudged it against a nerve. Every time I arched my back, it hurt, but the only way you can pitch is by arching your back.

I went to spring training with that condition and when I was pitching, I would be fine for three or four innings. But if I made one false move, it would pinch and I would have to stop. It would be okay after a half-hour's rest, and it so frustrated me that I finally donned a rubber pad for some support and stayed away from any workouts which affected that area of my back. But throughout my career I geared much of my exercise program to help my back problems as much as any other benefit which I derived.

If, when you place your hand between your back and the wall, there is more than a hand's worth of space, you have what is called a "lordic" or swayback posture or forward-tilted pelvis. If so, stretch the hip flexors using the *Back Stretch* exercise with one leg, and with both legs. Also strengthen the abdominal muscles by doing the *Pelvic Tilt* and the *Partial Sit-up* from our regular exercise program.

Let's look now at the *pelvis level*. The dominant side of an individual—your right if you are right-handed, and vice versa—can cause a slightly higher hip and lower shoulder on that side. To find out, stand against the wall and do the side-bend stretching exercise and see if you can reach farther down your leg on one side than the other. If you can, that hip probably is higher than the other. You also can eyeball it by looking in a mirror and checking very carefully the two sides of your body around your waist. On the side where the hip is higher there will be an additional fold of skin around your waist. The other side will seem flatter and slightly more elongated.

The side with the slightly higher hip will have tightness in the lateral trunk muscles, which prevented you from bending and reaching farther down your leg on the opposite side. Stretch the tight side by doing *Side Bends* to the opposite side and holding them for a 5-count. You also must strengthen the lateral hip muscles on the dominant side with *Side Leg Lifts* and work the other side with additional *Side Bends* to that side.

BODY MECHANICS

Body mechanics simply are the most efficient method to use your body mechanically to perform physical activity or work. That can mean sitting the right way, lying the right way or lifting the right way—things you do every day of your life.

But do you do them properly enough to avoid postural problems or an injury, slight or not so slight? Or to achieve maximum comfort? Let's look at the principles of good body mechanics and see how the body moves and how energy and force affect it.

(1) *Good Sitting Posture:* Includes keeping the upper back straight, maintaining the normal curve in the lower back, keeping the knees bent and slightly higher than the hips, keeping the arms supported; your buttocks flat on the seat; the pelvis not rotated backward or forward; and your feet flat on the floor.

(2) *Lying Position:* On your back, put a pillow under your head and one or two pillows under your knees.

(3) *On Your Side:* Curl up and put one pillow under your head and one between your knees.

(4) *On Your Abdomen:* Put a pillow beneath the abdomen and another under your ankles.

Here are some good points regarding proper body mechanics when movement is involved:

(1) *Pushing and Pulling:* Your aim when you push and pull is to keep your body in a good, stable position, with good alignment to prevent any back problems.

To *push* an object, face it and get a firm grip on its middle. Bend your elbows and keep them close to your sides. Be sure your pelvis is at the same level as the object's center and don't twist your back; change position if you must. Spread your feet to shoulder width, one a bit ahead of the other, and bend your knees, doing a pelvic tilt. Then begin pushing by shifting your body weight forward from your back foot to your front foot, keeping your arms rigid and close to the body. Keep your trunk straight and pelvis tilted, and keep the object moving to lessen the effects of inertia and friction.

To *pull* the object, assume the same position with the object as if you were pushing it, and start pulling by shifting your body weight backward from your front to back foot. Maintain your pelvic tilt and use the leg muscles instead of your arms. To really help your cause, use dollies, casters or rollers—and anything round that supports the weight of that object can be a roller—or get help from someone. If the object is flat on the ground, tilt it to reduce the amount of surface friction.

(2) *Stooping, Squatting, Kneeling:* If you learn how to do these properly, then you'll eliminate many of the dangers which lead to back problems. For example, lifting something by bending from the waist is bad for your back because of the stress on the small muscles of the back. Instead, bend with your legs, or stoop, or squat.

When you want to lift something from the floor, bend down from your hips and knees as if to squat, but not from the waist.

When stooping, squatting or kneeling, face the object from the front so you don't twist your back. Your feet should be at shoulder width with one foot slightly ahead of the other. Do a pelvic tilt and lower yourself by bending your knees, keeping your back upright as much as possible. Use those strong leg muscles which are firmly braced by the floor rather than your smaller back muscles.

(3) *Lifting and Carrying:* A prime cause of back injuries when done incorrectly. Begin by using your head—not to lift, but to figure out how to attack the problem. Decide if the object is too large or too heavy to be lifted by you alone. If so, can you get help? Should it be pushed...or slid...or pulled?

If you decide you can lift it, remember that your leg muscles—not those back muscles—will do the work after you assume the same kind of position in front of the object as before and lower yourself by bending your hips and knees—not at the waist! Grasp the object firmly in both hands and hold it as close to your body as possible near your pelvis. Stand up by lifting yourself and the object simply by straightening your knees; and maintain that pelvic tilt while you are carrying the object. To set it down, repeat the same process, again remembering to bend down with your legs rather than from your back.

Some other back-saving tips:

(1) If you are carrying a heavy object and need to turn around, don't twist at the waist, but move your feet to turn your entire body.

(2) If you need to work in one position, where you must reach up or reach down for a prolonged period of time, adjust your body level. If lower, bend to do the work; if higher, get a stool to raise your level.

(3) When getting into a car, particularly a small one, sit facing the door with both feet on the ground, and then swing them around into the car. Get out the same way.

If you do much of that lifting, pushing and pulling which I have just described, you may be ready for a meal. And just as there is a correct way to push and pull, there also is a correct way to approach your nutrition, as we'll see in the next chapter.

BODY BALANCE/GOOD POSTURE EXERCISES

POSTURAL EXERCISES	POSTURAL PROBLEM:			
	Forward Head/ Stiff Neck	Round Shoulders	Sway Back— Forward-Tilted Pelvis	High Hip
Chin Tuck	10–15X			
Neck Bend*	5X each way			
Reverse Two-Arm Hug*		5X		
Overhead Stretch*		5X each way		
Back Arm Reach—Palms Out*		5X		
Shoulder-Blade Pinch*		10–15X—hold 3 sec.		
Back Stretch*			5X each way	
Sprinter*			5X each way	
Pelvic Tilt*			5–10X	
Partial—Full Sit-up*			5–10X	
Side Bends*				15X to opp. side
Side Leg Lifts*				15X on same side

*Exercise movements have been explained in Chapters 2 and 3.

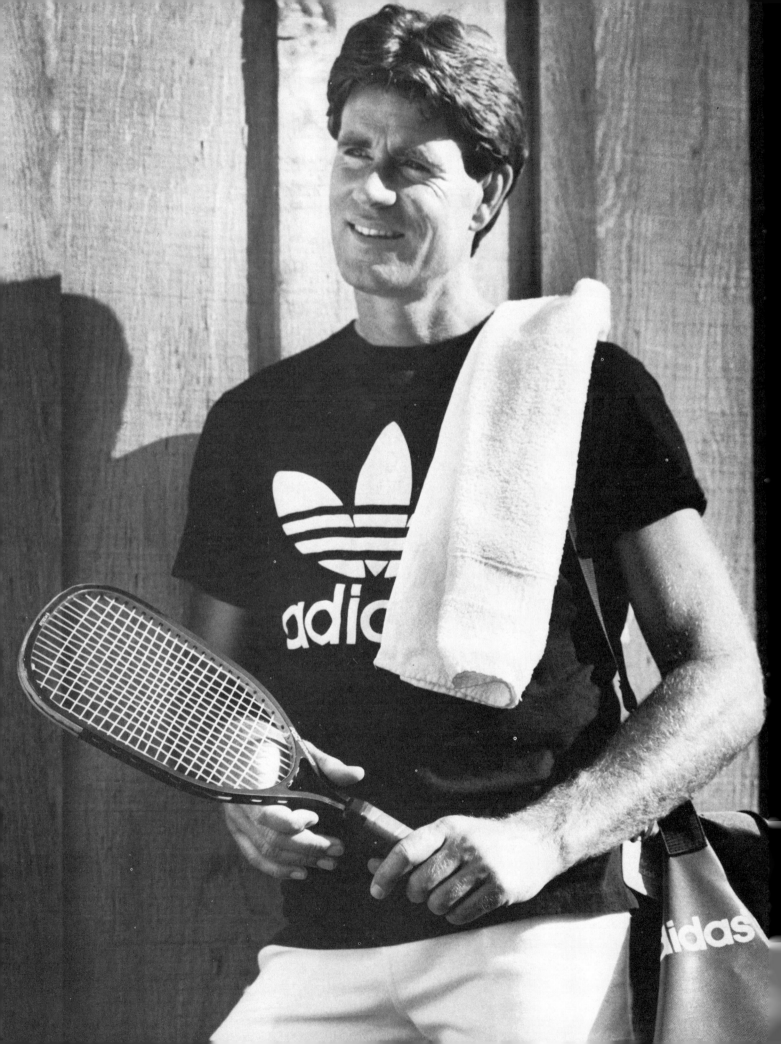

CHAPTER 5

NUTRITIONAL EDGE: BALANCING GOOD TIMES AND GOOD FOOD

Thus far, you've been doing quite a bit of work with your body, and a sound body, like a sound machine, doesn't run unless it has the correct amount of fuel.

Your fuel is what you eat.

Your fuel is what you eat, and that includes how much and how often.

This is an area where I can give you, from firsthand experience, the dos and don'ts—and particularly the don'ts, because the dietary life of most major-league ballplayers runs counter to nearly every sound nutrition principle ever laid down. Since most of their work is done at night and isn't finished until nearly midnight, professional ballplayers have a tendency to eat late, then sleep late the next day. Their lifestyle and eating habits are devoid of concern for nutritional balance.

Much of what I learned about sound nutrition—and I gathered as much documented information on the subject as I could because I felt it was integral to prolonging my career—showed me that I had to improve my nutritional habits. I was never a compulsive eater, but a meal wasn't really a meal for me early in my major-league career unless I polished it off with pie à la mode.

From the beginning, I ate pancakes before I pitched, and in my first full season as a starter back in 1965 I won four games in a row with this eating regimen. I lost the fifth game in Kansas City after we had made an early-morning flight from the West Coast and I missed my breakfast—not that pancakes really had much to do with it, but all ballplayers are creatures of habit (and superstition in one form or another). Then I won four games in a row with that pre-game meal. Soon the players were checking to see if I'd had my pancakes before I pitched. It wasn't long before they started calling me Jim "Pancakes" Palmer, and for the rest of my career I had the nickname "Cakes." But I really was storing carbohydrates before the practice became popular. Gone are pre-game meals for football where only steak and potatoes are served. Now teams feature pancakes, scrambled eggs, fish, green vegetables and, for those who think it helps, steak. A doctor once told me that the ideal pre-game meal was a bowl of oatmeal. I can just imagine the reaction from a group of athletes if that was all they could eat.

When I was away from home with the Orioles, I ate two light meals and one full meal a day, even on the days when I pitched. I often rose early and had a light breakfast, then ate my main meal in mid-afternoon, whether or not I was going to pitch that night.

However, earlier in my career it was what I consumed after a game that was wrong. Playing so many night games, home and away, players' eating habits can get turned around. Some still have a big meal following a night game and many of them are always fighting a weight problem. I never liked going to bed with a full stomach, so I used to order an omelet, or have a couple of scrambled eggs, until I found that eating too many eggs simply wasn't a good idea. Then I switched to a very light meal, something no heavier than fruit, a green salad or a bowl of soup.

Having gone through this for so long, I can sympathize with those of you who do a great deal of traveling and must try to keep an eating regimen close to the one you follow at home. It isn't easy, but it isn't impossible. Every menu contains something that you can eat within moderation, and if a dinner includes fried potatoes, for example, ask to substitute a vegetable or perhaps a baked potato. Tell the waiter or waitress not to bring bread to your table if you are eating alone. Or eat bread without butter. For dessert, order fresh fruit, or pass dessert altogether. If you get hungry late at night, instead of going into a coffee shop and ordering a piece of cake, ask for a piece of fruit.

I didn't vary that routine much when we played at home, except that I always had breakfast and then my main meal before going to the ball park. After the game, I had a piece of fruit or a light snack before going to bed. I did it to keep my weight at a level which was beneficial to my work, and as I got older and could see the dangers posed by putting on weight, I became more careful than ever, both in my eating habits and in my exercise schedule.

Stay light and strong to compensate for the aging factor.

You must make a concession to your body if you want to stay and look fit, particularly when you hit the age of thirty, when your metabolism may begin to slow down and your calorie burning isn't as intense. I boiled matters down to a logical sequence for me: I wanted to play as long as possible (and I lasted till I was thirty-eight years old), but if I consumed as much food as I had before I was thirty, that could mean as much as ten or fifteen additional pounds during the last eight years of my career. Do that and my natural skills would begin to erode quickly, I felt, and so would my reflexes because they would have to carry that extra weight. Stay light and strong and I could compensate for the aging factor. There is little doubt that this was a key reason why I was able to play for so long.

I will grant that as you get older and pay strict attention to your diet and work on your exercise program, you may have to be more attentive to your calorie intake and you're likely to feel frustrated because you don't seem to be getting much of a payoff. You're really working to stay even, so you must be more conscientious and not take anything for granted.

The key obviously is to eat a balanced diet and to be certain that your body receives all of the food properties needed to sustain its health. That requires some knowledge and planning, so I am going to outline just what properties the foods you eat do contain, and how they can help you. If you know what is involved in the three meals you consume each day, you will be better able to plan them from a nutritional standpoint and fully complement the exercise training programs which we already have outlined.

Proper exercise, coupled with proper diet, is the only course to follow. You will understand more about this as you read on, beginning with the most watched item in our diet—calories.

CALORIES

Simply stated, calories are a measure of the energy available to our bodies from the food we eat. This energy is required for the body to carry out all of its basic functions (digestion, breathing, maintenance of muscle tone, regulation of body temperature, etc.) for growth and for physical activity.

That's the good news.

On the other hand, of the many nutrients necessary for good health, only a few provide calories; thus, weight control is the balancing factor … what you put in as calories versus what you expend as energy. To maintain your weight, your ins should equal your outs; to lose, your outs must exceed your ins; and to gain, your ins must be greater than the outs.

Here's a good guide: The number of calories you must consume to maintain your weight can be figured by multiplying your weight in pounds by 15—if you are moderately active. Thus, if you weigh 170 pounds, you require approximately 2,550 calories per day to hold that weight. If you consume fewer, you'll lose pounds; if you consume more, you'll gain.

Now, this is not a hard and fast rule because there are cases of people who have consumed less than the supposed number required to maintain their weight and still have *gained*—and vice versa. Generally, 3,500 calories equals one pound of fat, so to lose a pound per week you must have a 3,500-calorie deficit, either in less intake or more exercise. Don't get greedy (pardon the pun) on the weight-loss routine: One or two pounds per week is plenty. Remember, it may have taken years to put on those pounds, so you can't expect to lose them all at one time.

On a personal note, I am not a counter of calories, but I am certainly aware of their presence and if I know I'm going to have a big meal with all the trimmings—say, at Thanksgiving—I watch my eating carefully before and after the large meal.

I do believe that if people counted their calories and watched their salt intake, they would be amazed. I saw it firsthand with Jim Weisner, who was the visiting team's clubhouse attendant in Minnesota. He drank a lot of diet soda and I guess he watched, or at least thought he did, his diet, yet he had a 38-inch waist. A couple of seasons ago, when I saw him for the first time since the previous year, he was down to a 32-inch waist.

"What did you do?" I asked him.

"I stopped drinking diet sodas and cut out salt on my food." Jim was becoming aware of exactly what he was eating and its effect on his body and weight.

"In addition," he went on, "I started walking around the ball park every day. Pretty soon I was walking around five times a day, then I ran around one time and walked around four times, and after a while I got to the point where I was running five miles a day. I lost six inches in my waist, and I look better and feel better about myself.

"But all I really did was watch what I was eating and get into an exercise program."

Stay with it, I told him. When you make the decision to watch your intake and couple that with exercise, you must also be willing to pay the price of staying with it.

FATS

Fats are the body's stockpile of fuel. Not all fat is bad—some is essential to everyone's diet. It is estimated that 42 percent of our national diet is made up of fat, whereas 10 to 20 percent is reasonable and desirable if you exercise regularly. That is cause to check on just how much you are ingesting each day.

Fat, as a condition, has become Public Enemy No. 1 for those who wish to regain their attractive selves, but fat, as a substance for bodily well-being, has positive functions, which include:

(1) A source of energy
(2) A source of essential fatty acid
(3) A carrier of fat-soluble vitamins

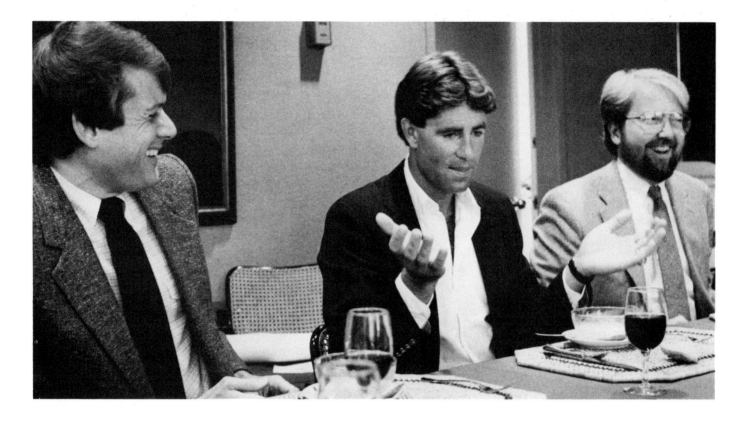

You have heard much about the pros and cons of saturated and polyunsaturated fats, and how they relate to what has become a dietary buzzword, "cholesterol."

Saturated fats are believed to raise blood cholesterol levels and, if these levels become too high, can lead to heart disease. These saturated fats are solid at room temperature and can be found in such foods as butter, cream, beef fat; and in hydrogenated fats such as solid vegetable shortening; other sources include palm oil, coconut oil and cocoa butter.

Polyunsaturated fats are found generally in liquid vegetable oils, such as corn oil and safflower oil. The good news here is that polyunsaturates tend to lower blood cholesterol levels.

And the million-dollar word: *Cholesterol.* This is a fatlike substance produced by our body as well as being found in many of the foods we eat. Now, some is necessary for many bodily functions, but excess levels are associated with a higher risk of heart disease and atherosclerosis. The chief culprits include egg yolks and organ meats such as liver. It's a good idea to have your cholesterol level checked when you have an annual or biannual physical, particularly if you are middle-aged.

One last thing: The sources of fats include such obvious products as butter, margarine, oils and fat which is not trimmed from fresh meat or is within the meat itself; plus foods such as nuts and seeds, avocados and poultry skin, the latter being the reason so many nutritionists advise skinning that chicken breast or leg before you cook it.

PROTEIN

Protein—the name is derived from a Greek word that means "primary importance"—is essential for our diets, particularly for the formation, growth, maintenance and repair of all bodily tissues. It supplies almost all of the nitrogen which the body requires, nitrogen which can *only* be supplied by the food which we eat.

Recent research shows that while protein is the main solid constituent of muscle tissue, and is used by the body to maintain muscle growth, it *does not* serve as an efficient energy fuel; in fact, it's downright inefficient in this function. Thus, the old saw about having to eat a big steak before playing football was really off base. If anything, a steak-fed football team may have had its performance hindered, not enhanced.

My own diet consists of about 10 to 20 percent protein, which is the percentage advocated by many nutritionists.

Proteins are made up of amino acids. Eight of the twenty amino acids are essential, and those which our body cannot produce must come from our diet. Animal products, such as meat, have all the essential amino acids which we need, and in the proper amounts which our body requires. But plant proteins do not, hence the need to combine different foods such as beans and rice, to gain those necessary numbers. When good nutritionists put together a ''balanced diet,'' that is one of the considerations in advising certain combinations of foods.

CARBOHYDRATES

Carbohydrates, or ''carbos'' as they have come to be popularly called since the marathon craze has taken over the land (as in ''loading up with carbos''), are the third essential nutrient, and are usually the largest component of your diet. Their major function is to provide energy in the form of glucose, the body's preferred fuel. (The brain and central nervous system can only use glucose for energy.)

Simple sugars and starches are the two main types of carbohydrates. *Simple sugars* such as sucrose and sugar should be avoided because they provide calories but little nutrition. It is best to rely mainly on complex carbohydrates—whole-grain products, beans, legumes, all of which provide many other nutrients and fiber as well as supplying carbohydrates.

Our body uses carbohydrates in the following ways after they are eaten:

(1) They may be metabolized immediately for energy.

(2) They may be converted to glycogen and stored in the liver or muscle when intake exceeds the amount immediately needed. Glycogen is a reserve of carbohydrates which can be called upon

as a source of glucose when needed. Marathoners always are concerned about glycogen levels, hence they ''load up with carbos'' up to four hours before a race, to raise those levels as high as possible.

Periodic ridding of glycogen is dangerous because sudden depletion can cause numerous problems such as mood changes, altered sleep patterns and even ruptured muscle tissue. The safest bet is to keep your diet continually high in carbohydrates and to couple it with regular exercise.

(3) As with added calorie-producing nutrients, the intake that far exceeds the needs can be converted to fat and stored as such. You can increase your ability to store glycogen through regular exercise. Working out will deplete glycogen reserves, but if the workout is followed with a meal high in fiber, not absorbed by the body, and whole grains, the glycogen reserves will quickly be restored.

LIQUIDS

I cannot overstress the importance of drinking an adequate amount of liquids daily. Water is my favorite, one which I drink during dinner and which I prefer to soft drinks, wine, beer, and liquor. I always recommend it as a thirst quencher.

I like it best because it tastes good—and because it has a number of very important functions within the body's system. Beginning with the fact that it comprises about 70 percent of the body, it also is the principal solvent for other nutrients, carrying them to the tissues. While carrying away waste products, it is the medium for most bodily chemical reactions; and it regulates body temperature. At rest, about one-quarter of your excess body heat is eliminated by means of water evaporation in the lungs and at the skin's surface. In hot weather and during strenuous exercise, much more water is evaporated in the same ways and is responsible for cooling you down.

With so much at stake, it is easy to see why we must replenish our body's water supply. How much water is enough? We eliminate a little over a quart per day in the form of urine, so that much, at least, must be replaced, which means six to eight glasses per day, and more in hot weather and during exercise.

I had to confront both situations when I pitched in the summertime in Baltimore, where the humidity can be as oppressive as the heat and cause dehydration much quicker than in less humid climates. I always made sure I drank plenty of water during the games I worked, and its importance is such that it has become the main ingredient of many diets. It is firmly fixed in my dietary regimen. One last thought: You *can* acquire a taste for water.

I drink three or four glasses at dinner alone. In fact, it was somewhat of a nuisance several years ago when a water shortage in New York City was the excuse for restaurants to stop serving water unless a customer requested it. I was used to having a glass of cold water as a pre-dinner drink, and I'd get some dirty looks from the waiters when I had to make a specific request for the first glass, and then for refills.

Hot weather and exercise require an increase in liquid consumption.

Hot weather and exercise also require an increase in consumption, and of course that goes against the old saw when I was growing up that when you played certain sports, such as football, you never took water during practice or a game lest you get stomach cramps. Doctors long since have found that the body needs liquid replenishment during these times, and I know that in football training camps, where drills are conducted in 80° and 90° temperatures, portable water carts are available for the players at all times.

One of the consequences of dehydration—when the body loses too much liquid during strenuous exercise—is muscle cramping. A natural thirst is nature's way of telling you it's time for a drink, but don't wait for that signal, particularly if you exercise strenuously and regularly. By the time you feel thirsty, your body may be too dehydrated to perform at full peak. Drink whether you're thirsty or not, and drink beyond feeling satiated during those strenuous periods.

One word to you long-distance or marathon runners: If you haven't already tried it, it's a good idea to splash water—or have it splashed—on the outside of you to aid your body's natural cooling process.

VITAMINS

Perhaps no other area of nutrition invites more dissension—and discussion—than the use of vitamin supplements. You probably heard about them from your parents during your earliest years. If you read the ingredient information on the food packages, you see vitamins listed; and you hear about certain products which give you the "suggested daily minimum requirements." Magic is accorded to some products, bodily healing attributed to others, and absolute prevention of anything from the common cold to leprosy, or so it would seem, as a benefit from taking still other vitamins.

What are these so-called elixirs of life?

The term "vitamin" was first used by a biochemist named Casimir Funk in 1912 to describe a substance both vital for life and containing nitrogen (amines). Scientists have since discovered the qualities and benefits of many different vitamins. Here is a list of the most important ones:

Vitamin A: Aids night vision, or seeing any time when light is limited. It is necessary for normal tissue growth, and it helps to keep moist tissues healthy, especially passages of the nose and throat. A deficiency is marked by dry, cracked skin and dim vision. Vitamin A is abundantly available in vegetables such as carrots, pumpkins, broccoli, tomatoes, turnips, spinach and certain tropical fruits such as papayas, canteloupes and mangoes. In general, vegetables rich in Vitamin A are identified by the color: orange, dark green, or yellow. Vitamin A is fat-soluble, not water-soluble, meaning that it can be stored in the body. That is why taking supplements may be dangerous, and an overdose can be highly toxic.

B-complex Vitamins: The B-complex is

made up of many different vitamins. Let's make it easy—here are some of the general functions and the foods in which they can be found:

First, the word "complex" in B-complex gives a clue that B-complex vitamins are complicated and wide-ranging in their function. They are a group of elements necessary for releasing energy in the body, and they work with enzymes to enable protein, fat and carbohydrates to be metabolized. Some B-complex vitamins aid in preventing anemia. They occur in varying amounts in the following foods: beans, whole grains, brown rice, wheat germ, green leaf vegetables, peas, lentils, brewer's yeast, meats (especially organ meats) and dairy products.

An excess of the B-complex is generally thought to pass out of the body, and overdosing does not appear to pose the risks that can occur with overconsumption of vitamins A and D.

Vitamin C, or Ascorbic Acid: Vitamin C helps to heal wounds, prevent infections, form bones and teeth and strengthen some body tissues. Taking supplements of Vitamin C also is said to hold down the incidence of colds, but it is not a cure-all. Actually, Vitamin C may make you feel better when you have a cold, but it cannot prevent you from catching one.

Vitamin C is water-soluble, meaning you must replenish it regularly, and since it's unstable in the presence of heat and oxygen, it is best to eat Vitamin-C-rich foods raw—as fresh as possible. These include citrus fruits, tomatoes, strawberries, raw peppers, raw spinach, watercress and potatoes.

A deficiency of Vitamin C is marked by the symptoms of "scurvy:" loosening teeth, bleeding gums and very painful joints.

Vitamin D: Provided by three main sources: milk (Vitamin D is added by most milk manufacturers); bony fish such as sardines, salmon and tuna; and sunlight. (Sunlight doesn't contain Vitamin D, but its effect causes the body to metabolize it.) It will help to produce strong bones and teeth; it enables the body to use calcium and phosphorus, which are essential to proper skeletal growth. A deficiency is marked by various bone and spinal deformities, causing a disease called "rickets," whose symptoms include bowlegs and "pigeon breast"—deformity of the chest.

Vitamin E: Another controversial vitamin for which great claims have been made, such as promoting sexual stamina and potency, increased longevity, and a safeguard against any number of diseases. Don't buy the claims because all are unproven!

But Vitamin E *has* been proven to be an antioxidant and it helps to prevent the breakdown of bodily tissues. It occurs naturally in a number of foods already mentioned, particularly those providing Vitamin A and the B-complex. Some particularly rich Vitamin E foods include whole grains, wheat germ, green leafy vegetables and vegetable oils.

Vitamin Supplements: My only advice here is to consult a doctor or nutritionist if you believe you are still vitamin-deficient. Don't walk into a health store and start loading up on supplements, and don't depend solely on the advice of those who sell the supplements. Proper guidance is a must because there can be toxic effects from excessive amounts.

MINERALS

If you eat adequate amounts of vitamin-rich foods, you'll probably get adequate doses of iron, calcium, phosphorus, magnesium, iodine, fluoride, sodium, potassium and other "trace" elements. All are essential in varying ways, but all are needed in very small amounts. As with vitamins—and this is why I believe you needn't worry about supplements—if you follow a healthy diet, eating a variety of foods prepared so that vitamin and mineral loss is minimized, you probably will be assured of getting what you require.

PUTTING THIS TOGETHER

This seems like a lot to understand and apply. But one of the simplest ways to insure that you are getting the necessary vitamins and minerals is to eat foods from the four basic food groups.

Foods with similar nutrient content may be grouped together. There are four nutrient-based food groups—milk, meat, fruit-vegetable and grain.

Here are the main nutrients and foods included in each group:

Milk Group: These include milk and dairy products, and I begin my list with skim milk, the only kind I drink. Two servings per day from this group are recommended: 1 cup of skim milk or low-fat yogurt and 1½ ounces of low-fat cheese. The only cheese product I use is Parmesan cheese, and this is part of the milk group. Also included, if you wish, would be 1 cup of pudding, 1¾ cups of ice cream and 2 cups of cottage cheese. Cheese can be considered as one serving in the milk group or in the meat group, but not in both simultaneously.

Meat Group: I eat hardly any red meat, a practice which most nutritionists endorse. And when you do, they insist, make it lean and eat only in small servings, not more than 4 to 6 ounces daily. But there are other products than red meat in this group, including veal, fish and shellfish; poultry; eggs; legumes such as dry beans, peas, lentils, peanuts and nuts.

Skin the poultry to remove much of the fat. Don't eat oily fish, or if you do, cut down the portion. I prefer my fish broiled. Water-packed fish is better than oil-packed any day.

Grain Group: Foods in this group supply carbohydrates, thiamin, iron and niacin, and include all grains such as barley, buckwheat, corn, oats, rice, rye and wheat—and the bread, breakfast cereals, grits, noodle and pasta products made from them.

You are better off relying on whole grains, with a minimum four servings per day. What is a serving? 1 slice of bread ... 1 cup of dry cereal ... ½ cup of cooked cereal, rice, pasta. You can increase the servings in this group proportionately with your calorie needs.

Fruit-and-Vegetable Group: Foods in this group supply Vitamins A and C, and include all fresh, canned, frozen and dried fruits and vegetables, except dried beans and peas. The latter, as we noted earlier, are in the Meat Group because they contain significant amounts of protein. Corn may be served as a vegetable; corn grits and meal are in the grain group.

Eating foods from this group requires a minimum of four servings daily—a serving being ½ cup of vegetables or juices, 1 full cup of raw fruit or vegetables and a common portion of fruit such as a medium-sized apple or banana. You also can increase this group proportionately with your individual needs.

There also is one other kind of food to be discussed—*junk food.*

Obviously, my advice on junk food is to stay away from it. You certainly have seen a great variety of worthy substitutes which are much better for your health.

I have plenty of firsthand experience with this kind of eating because baseball locker rooms seem to proliferate with it as post-game snacks or meals. Walk into a major-league dressing room and you find candy bars, fried foods, cold cuts, beer, sodas—all the things which don't really enhance your performance.

Major-league players get $46 per day in meal money, and for them there really is no excuse for not eating the proper foods. For several years I suggested to the Orioles management that they replace the junk food with fruit and nuts as a post-game snack, which would almost force the players to eat properly. I don't blame the players entirely because no one has ever taken the time to talk to them about the liabilities of junk food.

Selection of the proper foods is up to you. Conscientiously cut down on high-fat foods such as butter (and regular margarine is not better) and high-fat meat such as pork and beef. Eat fruit for dessert, or a fresh fruit compote for variety. The juices from the fruits provide their own tasty topping. And don't use salt because there will be more than sufficient quantities of sodium present in a diet based on the food groups we've just discussed. To enliven flavors, think in terms of pepper—I use it as a flavor in soup—lemon and lime juice, which is great for melon and as a salad dressing; garlic; onion; and herbs and spices.

When you purchase food, read the labels on packaged foods. You'll be surprised at the amount of salt and sugar listed in the ingredients. Avoid any product that has hidden salt and sugar, and in general think about preparing your meals from fresh ingredients instead of seeking pre-cooked or prepared foods. I do this whenever possible. It is

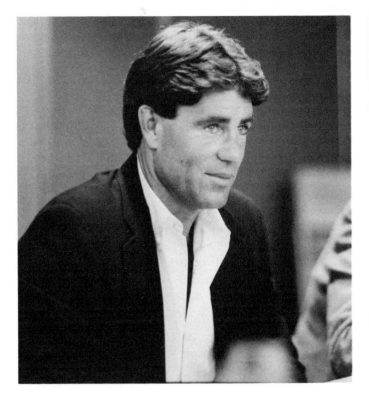

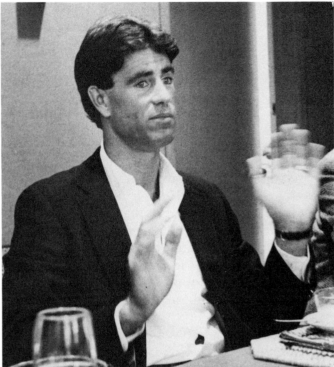

not difficult, and it is rather satisfying—as well as being eminently more nutritious.

Most of us, given the opportunity, like to take a turn around the kitchen, and once you begin and chalk up a few victories, the feeling becomes addictive. But before you prepare you must plan, and planning a meal around carbohydrates instead of around meat is a very good starting point. For instance, a meal of spaghetti and a low-fat sauce is a perfect example, and so is rice or beans as the basis of a meal.

When you cook, poach, steam, bake or broil your meat, fish and chicken.

When you cook, it is best to poach, steam, bake or broil your meat and fish (including chicken); stir-fry or steam vegetables, or, if possible, eat them raw. I prefer to defrost frozen things slowly and cook them so as to allow time for all of a food's ingredients to interact with each other. Friends who use a microwave oven—and I have one—say they are getting the same results, but I still prefer the old-fashioned method.

I offer this advice in full knowledge that many of you are single and must do the shopping, planning and preparation yourself, but that should not matter. How hard is it to stop on the way home from work and pick up a piece of fish or a chicken breast, or to take one from your freezer in the morning and allow it to thaw through the day? You can sauté it, or bake it in about 25 minutes, or broil it in even less time. You can marinade it in something of your choice and make it really delicious. To me, it's a copout to claim that you can't cook for one person. It's a matter of priorities, and that's what this book and its programs really are about. Do you want to feel better and look better, or do you just want to cop out and settle for a fast-food burger? You must be willing to make some effort.

For those of you who will use these programs to lose weight, the nutrition side is very important, particularly if you couple it with exercise which can accelerate the weight loss, rather than relying on diet alone. I am not suggesting ry-krisp and lettuce for weight loss; in fact, my motto is "Eat healthy and you will lose weight," because everything will be in the right proportions—the amount of your intake, the food properties and the balance.

I've done the diet routine with many of my friends and I know what they endure. In fact, when I went to Puerto Rico for two months to play winter ball in 1968, while rehabilitating myself after an arm injury, I dropped almost twenty pounds, though not consciously. The heat and humidity, plus the fact that most of the foods were pre-packaged and frozen imports which had little appeal, were natural incentives. And once I had the weight off, I felt so comfortable that I took great pains to keep it off. As I noted, that reduced weight helped to prolong my career, and that was a great incentive.

Spring training has always been a period of great temptation for ballplayers. While the object of the six weeks in Florida is to get your body and your baseball skills in order, the life is far from grueling. Practice runs about four hours a day until exhibition games begin, which leaves most of the afternoon and evening for casual pursuits. Even though soup and sandwiches were served at lunch every day, I never had a sandwich during two decades of spring training, but concocted a home-made brew instead. If I consumed it before going to practice, it held me through the day. It consisted of orange juice, grapefruit juice, milk, banana, some strawberries and an egg, all of which I mixed in a blender. Accompanied with a bowl of whole-grain cereal, it gave me all the energy I needed. I got protein from the egg, potassium from the banana and energy from the natural sugars in the other fruits and juices.

I'd buzz off to practice for four hours and come home and play a couple of games of tennis and perhaps go swimming for a while. Rarely did I feel a need to eat, and if I did, I grabbed a piece of fruit or a cup of soup in the clubhouse before my tennis match.

A conscious weight-loss program coupled with exercise can certainly speed the weight-loss process. You need both to achieve your ends. As I have emphasized, it will take some will-power and

none of us are too naive to realize that you may deviate from your new routine simply because the temptation is so overpowering. I don't see anything fatal in having a hamburger once in a while; no one is perfect, and you don't want to follow a course that makes daily living a grueling ordeal.

A friend of mine is an ageless Hollywood stuntman named Ted Grossman who keeps himself in fantastic physical condition and is particularly careful about what he eats. That included going without sweets—no ice cream, no cookies—for almost a year. But when I saw him last year, he said, "You won't believe what happened to me when I was visiting San Francisco. I walked past this cookie store and something snapped. I guess my body couldn't stand it any longer. I went in and bought a baker's dozen of chocolate-chip macadamia cookies"—my favorites as well—"and I ate every one."

Of course he felt guilty about this and he went back "on the wagon" once that craving was satisfied. From time to time he gives in, but an occasional dalliance with a forbidden sweet is okay. But two days of dalliance a week will never help you. Fight it until you begin to see some weight loss and then the incentive to resist will grow stronger.

One final tip: If you need to lose weight, rely more on low-calorie fruits and vegetables from that food group; if you need to gain, rely more on the higher-calorie grain products.

Alcohol can severely dehydrate the body.

And one final caveat—regarding alcohol and the use of caffeine. I realize that you may be in a lifestyle that includes many social obligations, even as part of your work routine—cocktail parties, business lunches and dinners, receptions, as well as your own special social needs.

If you're looking for a way out here, forget it. Remember, we have talked about moderation in our intake, and this also applies to alcohol consumption. If you have one or two glasses of wine with dinner or at a social function, that should be okay. You should know your own capacity, but if you feel you still need something more to drink, go back to our old standby—water or club soda, which may appear "more sociable." Again, it brings will-power—I prefer the term "won't-power"—into play. But you must make up your mind that you are also changing your lifestyle when you take on programs such as these, and a reduced alcoholic intake is one of the changes.

The benefits to society aside, if you feel you must succumb to social pressure to drink, then I think you should look into a mirror and examine what you really think of yourself.

I am not moralizing. I drink an occasional glass of wine; I've never been a beer person; and I acquired a particular distaste for whiskey when I was a kid and used to fix my parents a scotch-and-water every night before dinner. I'd stir their drinks with my finger, and after I had licked it a few times, I found the taste very bitter. I never got over it.

I do know that drinking beer and whiskey will put on weight, though there are doctors who recommend that if a person is in a stressful position, a drink after work helps him to relax. Maybe so—that is a medical opinion. I've never had to survive under such conditions. But I do know that alcohol can severely dehydrate the body and, in even moderate amounts, attack vital organs such as the heart, liver and kidneys.

I don't drink coffee, either, and only a very occasional cup of tea, mostly iced tea, because of the caffeine content. Some nutritionists advocate the occasional use of caffeine because of its undeniable stimulatory effect, but in the same moderation as having just one glass of wine. As a rule, it probably is safer to limit your consumption of coffee to not more than two cups a day. Decaffeinated coffee gives you more leeway, and now even restaurants are serving it brewed. Soft drinks now feature brands without caffeine, and tea also is manufactured with the caffeine removed. You can't go wrong following that course.

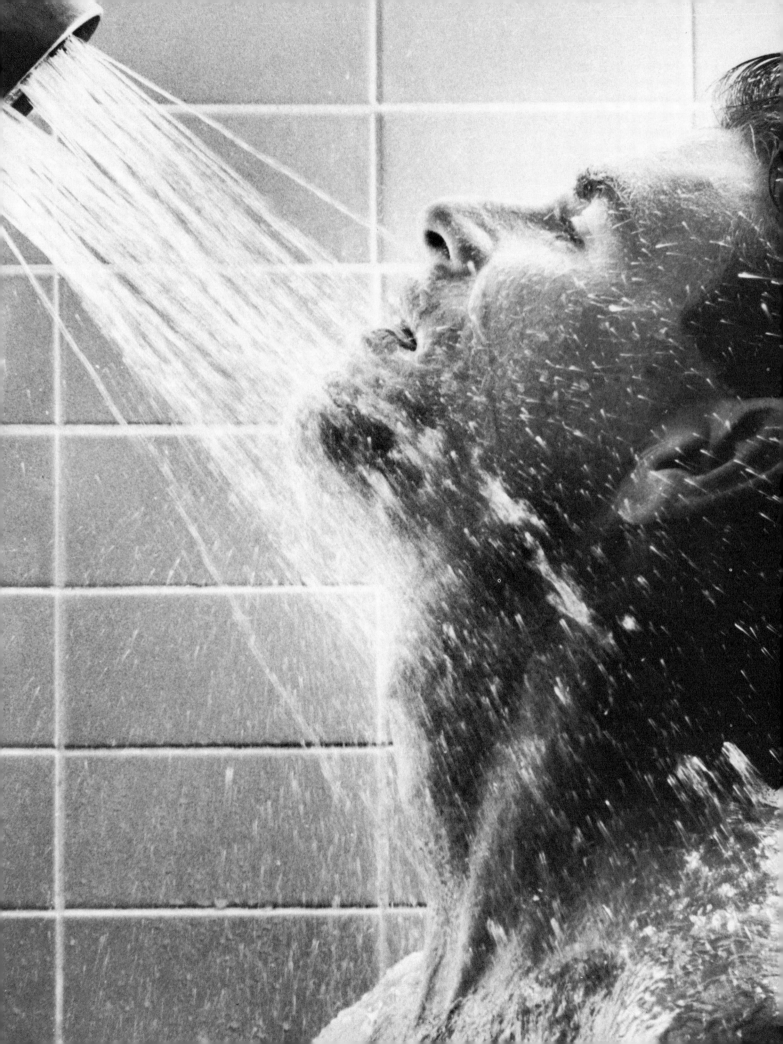

CHAPTER 6

THE PERSONAL TOUCH: HAIR AND SKIN CARE

We have discussed how best to get your body into shape and keep it that way. But what about the outward appearance of that body? It really is self-defeating to pour so much effort into streamlining yourself if you don't finish the job by looking good, smelling good and then dressing so that the entire package is worthy of admiration.

We'll discuss some ideas on wearing apparel in the next chapter because before we ever get to donning our clothes we must have something worthwhile to cover. And "worthwhile" in this chapter means showing off your skin to its best advantage, including those times when you are tanned, and then complementing it with a hair style that tells those around you that you have taken special care to present a first-class product.

Today more than ever, most men are acutely aware of how they look (if you weren't, you wouldn't have purchased this book). You need only to walk into the locker room of the Orioles or any other professional sports team, where a cross-section of male America spends a great deal of their time, to witness the sundry ways in which men groom themselves ... from the very fastidious (I guess I fell into the category because I was always conscious of my appearance) to the quick shower-and-scram guys who prefer more of the au-naturel look.

Everyone has his own unique look, something which is God-given and with which we all must cope for the rest of our lives. Men's bodies come in all types and sizes, and so do their looks. Some people consider me a handsome male, and I dare say that you consider yourself the same way.

How do we complement and enhance those attributes? How do we take care of the only face we ever will have, one that will change in appearance as we get older, but which will always be the focus of attention for anyone with whom we are in contact?

No matter what we do, we can't escape the fact that everything begins with the skin, which really is a seamless covering for that marvelous package called the human body. The outer layer, or the epidermis, is our protective covering, and its outer layer is composed of dead cells which are daily disposed of through washing or friction. They are continually replenished from the deepest part of the epidermis, where new cells are formed and begin their rise to the top, ultimately to be discarded in the same process.

Beneath this layer of skin is another, called the "dermis," which really is a feeding ground that nourishes the outer layer from its oil-producing and sweat glands and hair follicles. Those glands, called "sebaceous" because of their steady supply of "sebum," an oily-fatty substance which lubricates and protects the skin's outermost layer, come to the root of our discussion here.

Dry skin indicates that not enough natural oil is being produced.

How they work in your particular body determines whether you have dry or oily skin. Dry skin indicates that not enough natural oil is being produced, or that it isn't being produced fast enough to properly lubricate the skin's outer layer and replenish the oil being removed in cleansing.

Obviously, the opposite is true with oily skin—too much sebum is being produced.

Regardless of which type you may have—and I'll suggest shortly how best to cope with each problem—skin is only healthy when it is clean, and that means using some kind of cleanser.

As my schedule of in-person appearances expanded over the last several years, I took pains to seek the best advice on how best to present a clean look, and this is what I have found:

There are really three types of skin cleansers: *"true" soap,* which is a combination of water, sodium compounds, fatty acids and various oils; *detergent cleansers* made up of chemicals which replace the natural ingredients found in soap; and *creams,* such as cold cream, which act by liquifying on warm skin and then loosening dirt and other skin debris. Some detergent cleansers can be harsh; still,

they leave less of a residue on the skin and can be the most effective cleansers for men with oily skin. Creams tend to leave more of a film on the skin than true soap.

Thus, if you tend to have dry skin, as I do, then you don't want to oil your face to a high gloss, which simply attracts dirt, but to make sure that you hydrate—combine water and the cleansing ingredients—your skin regularly. It is true that a faint film of oil left by a cream can prevent water from evaporating quickly from dead skin cells if it is applied to slightly damp skin. But dry skin needs frequent washing to remove the dirt attracted by that film.

How to do that?

I use a facial soap which is almost pure, but I don't spend a lot of time massaging it into my skin because I don't want an excess drying effect. I'll also sometimes use a deodorant soap for the rest of my body, but I have been told by those who deal in the various body scents that a deodorant soap lessens the need for an after-bath spray or roll-on deodorant because it already has begun to do the job. So if you prefer the scent of a deodorant, then the pure soap may be for you.

I would say that the bottom line really is to use a cleanser that will remove as much oil and dirt as possible from the skin without damaging or irritating it. I compensate with an after-wash moisturizer.

Now, as I promised, here is advice on how to cope with cleansing dry or oily skin. For the former, cleanse your face thoroughly so as not to trap old oil and dirt with the water when you apply a moisturizer. Towel your face lightly, leaving it slightly damp, which is the water you'll be trapping to hydrate your skin. Apply a very thin film of moisturizer and massage lightly into the skin. One caveat here: It is particularly important at day's end to cleanse your face thoroughly if you have used a moisturizer.

If your skin is oily, wash it only with true soap.

If your skin is oily, wash it only with true soap. You can use an astringent such as an after-

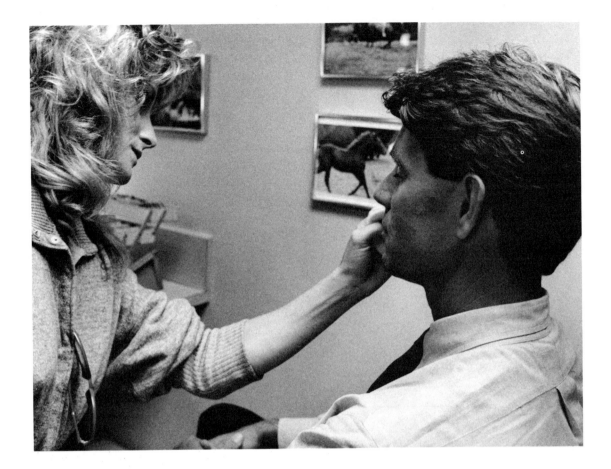

shave lotion or rubbing alcohol to speed up evaporation, but don't overdo. After using an astringent, you can apply a light moisturizer, but if you don't want to bother with that, you still should be sure to wash your face more than twice a day to cleanse and rehydrate it.

Since many of us shave after we have showered, bathed or washed our faces, we often interrupt the moisturizing process to mow away that stubble. I prefer a "wet shave" because it simply feels cleaner, smoother and more comfortable, both while I'm doing it and when I have finished. I always have been careful to first wet my face with water and then apply a shaving cream to hold that water; they work together to soften my beard so my razor can do the job cleanly and comfortably. I've known guys who use only water, or perhaps the soap they have used to clean their body, and do a very good job ... no nicks, no runs, no errors. If you're that tough, fine. But, regardless, you should rinse your face completely

and pat it dry, though leaving it a little moist. Now is a good time to apply moisturizer because shaving off the top layer of skin cells tends to dehydrate the skin quickly. And if you wish to use an after-shave lotion, my best recommendation is to be sure that it's an emollient. The stinging, astringent lotions really do nothing but further damage a dry skin.

For those who prefer electric shavers—remember they are only effective on dry beards—the only moistening can be a pre-electric shaving lotion, which, as an astrigent, will cause rapid drying of the skin and beard. This is particularly apt for shaving just after you've washed your face. And, like the wet shave, the electric mower also has rid your face of its top layer of skin, so the use of a moisturizer may be just as necessary.

Don't reach for those clothes just yet. Because you may wish to cap your ablutions with some scent, either a cologne or a body lotion. It used to be that men would slap on some after-shave lotion

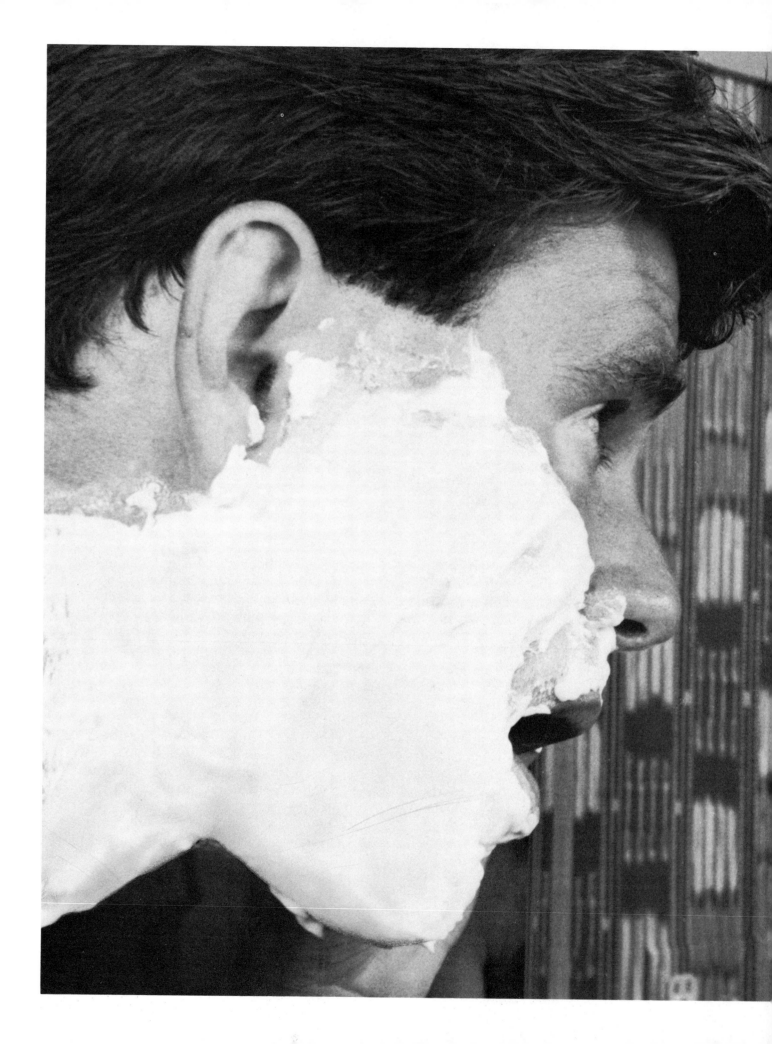

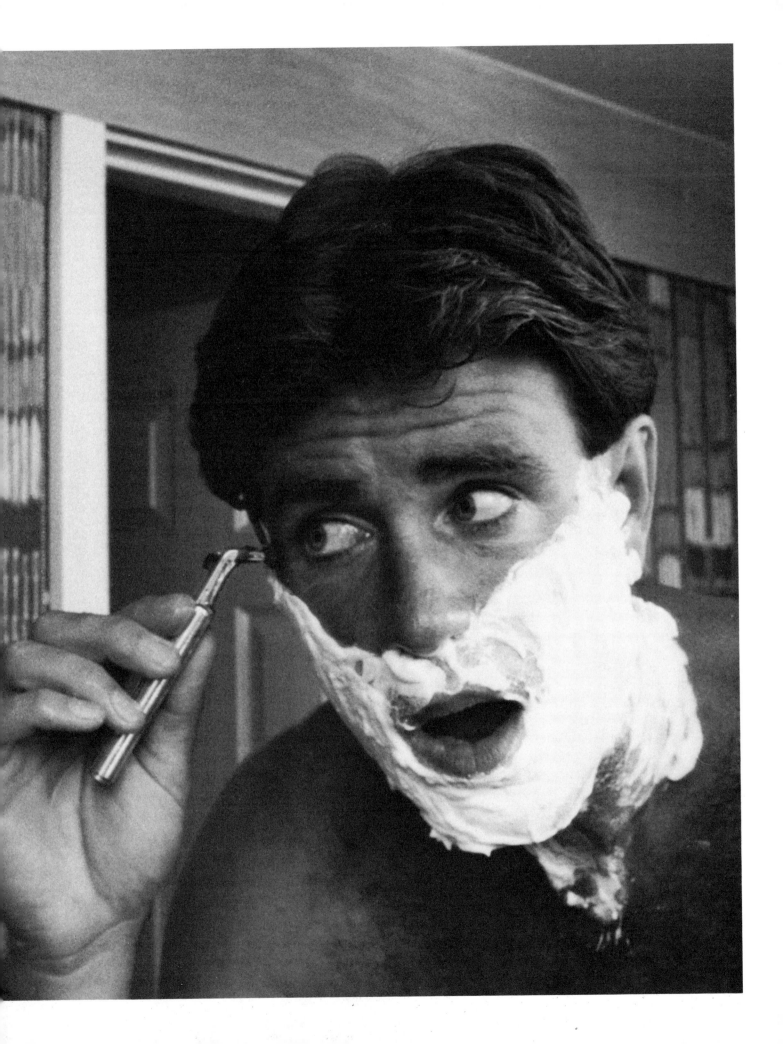

and allow that to carry them, but in recent years they have found that there is just as much to be gained by utilizing other areas of the body with some very pleasing, yet subtle, effects. I know it has shocked some of the older former players who walked into our locker room and saw young players using blow dryers and rubbing themselves with scented lotions. They just shook their heads and walked away, and within one frame of action there was the true essence of the generation gap.

Yet I have heard some of them remark that the routine is to be appreciated, and I heartily agree. My kids are always buying me colognes and after-shave lotions for my birthday, though I'm finicky about what I wear—and thank goodness they are. But then, why shouldn't we be? After all, the scent which we wear is really our signature, the same as a woman's perfume, something that is distinctly us. My girls, both teenagers who have become very aware of scents for a woman, often come in and use my Chaps for their perfume because they prefer its fragrance.

But finding what is right is not always easy, and often it's a trial-and-error process that may be resolved by the approval of your wife or girlfriend or a positive reaction from those around you.

I was shopping for some lotion at a store near my home in Baltimore one day, and two men were nearby looking over the assortment of colognes and body lotions. When I picked my brand off the shelf, I could see the men, who obviously had recognized me, watching closely, and as I walked past them, one said, "Well, if it's good enough for Jim Palmer, then it's good enough for me." And he bought the same brand.

I can appreciate his dilemma because I would not go up to a fragrance counter and have the clerk spray the various scents along the underside of my wrist so as to do some comparison sniffing, except perhaps if my girls were along and insisted on getting something that instant.

What this boils down to is that there is no hard and fast rule about choosing a scent, except to find the one you like and then use it sparingly. And don't—please don't—ever use a strong-smelling deodorant along with a different but equally strong-smelling cologne. If you use a deodorant, make sure it's neutral, or odorless.

There is no hard and fast rule about choosing a scent.

There is one more area regarding the skin which needs some discussion because it has become something of a national obsession with so many people—getting a suntan. No longer do we wait for the summer, or two weeks of winter vacation in the tropics. There are tanning parlors in cities and sun lamps in our homes as well as the natural process on ski slopes. But regardless of where we try it, we cannot escape the fact that our skin not only covers the body but also protects internal organs from the sun's harmful rays. It does so by producing a dark skin pigment which absorbs those rays, called melanin.

Dermatologists claim, and I have to agree, that there is no such thing as a "healthy" tan. Your skin colors in the sun because it is desperately trying to protect itself from damaging ultraviolet rays. Overexposure to the sun not only leads to dryness and wrinkles but the sun's rays can damage the skin's DNA, with possible skin cancer as the result.

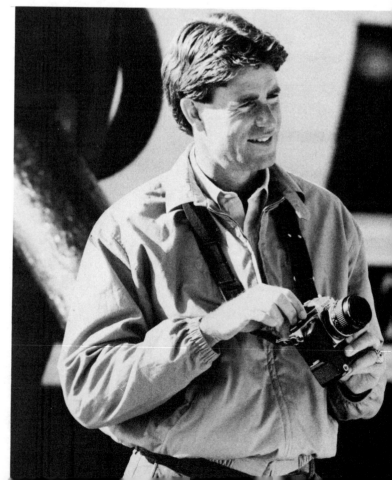

I tan very easily, and since many of my business interests take me to the sun belt at all times of the year, I have a constant tan. But I have been very careful, ever since my early days in baseball, to follow a set of procedures which do the utmost to safeguard my skin. If I stay out in the sun six or eight hours, and regardless of whether I have been in the sun a month or five days, I will get a sunburn.

Ballplayers find that out very early in their careers when they come to spring training and are out-doors each day for three or four straight hours when the sun is at its peak. You always see players who have come from colder winter climates with some kind of protective covering around their necks to shield themselves from that constant exposure until their skin has tanned enough to absorb it. There simply is no place to hide on the practice field.

I appreciated their dilemma last year when I went to Hawaii for a vacation without having had much exposure to the sun. For the next nine days I sought whatever shade I could find on the beach. Normally, I prefer to be active on the beach, either surfing or playing Frisbee or volleyball, or even walking, rather than lying there reading or just exposing my body to the sun.

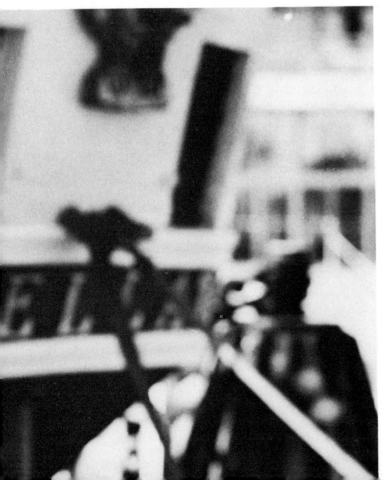

I try to get my skin gradually accustomed to its tanning process, and when I do, I always use a sunscreen tanning lotion, which I will discuss in greater detail in just a moment. But the best advice I ever received in trying to tan without a protective lotion was to avoid exposure between eleven a.m. and three p.m., when the sun's rays are most damaging. Instead, if you tend to be light-skinned and don't use a sunscreen lotion, then limit your first exposure to 15 minutes, your second to 20, third to 30, by which time you'll begin to see and feel what is the best process to follow.

But with the emergence of the sunscreens, it really makes little sense not to use one from the outset, on the beach or on the slopes. Each of the sunscreens is numbered according to how easily you burn and how long you wish to remain in the sun. For example, if you burn after 15 minutes exposure but you want to be out in the sun for two and a half hours, or 150 minutes, with the same degree of safety, the appropriate Sun Protective Factor (SPF) for you is 10, or 150 divided by 15. Many dermatologists recommend an SPF of 15 or higher, and I subscribe to that advice.

There are screens with even higher numbers, and a dermatologist whose advice I sought about this subject told me of someone who had been marooned on a raft but, because he'd had the proper screen application, wasn't seriously burned. He said a sunscreen can be worn in the water for 6 to 8 hours without losing its effectiveness.

Those who tan easily are not exempt from the dangers of overexposure.

Sunscreen preparations come in three types: those which absorb the sun's rays; those which reflect the rays; and those which do both. Those which reflect the rays are probably the safest because they completely block out the sun, like a No. 15, which of course means tanning will be almost impossible. I use Sundown No. 8, which is manufactured by Johnson & Johnson, because it allows an easy and gradual tan. Once I get the tan I want, then I'll use a lower sunscreen so I'll get some moisturizing and still screen the sun's ultraviolet rays.

However, you must determine what sunscreen strength is correct for your skin and tanning objectives. For those who tan easily, you are not exempt from the dangers of overexposure. For those who are fair-skinned, baking in the sun without taking necessary precautions is virtually suicidal and just invites excruciating pain and misery, to say nothing of dashed dreams for further tanning and a comfortable vacation.

The friends who accompanied me to Hawaii for that vacation last year prepared their skin with some sessions in a tanning parlor. Three visits did it for them, so that, with the proper precautions under the Hawaiian sun, they were out for long periods of time and were not bothered at all, while I spent much of the day hiding in the shade. But I believe that any such artificial tanning process, to be beneficial, requires proper supervision and advice.

HAIR CARE

Hair, like skin, comes in two varieties—dry and oily, caused by the production of those same sebaceous glands. I pretty much fall in between the two, with none of the flaking problems of dry scalp and none of the greasy qualities from too much oil.

However, as an athlete who exercised pretty vigorously throughout the year, I always was faced with the problem of when and how to shampoo so as not to allow all of the waste products generated by my physical regimen to accumulate and take away the qualities from what I know is a pretty good head of hair.

I have found that antidandruff shampoos work fine for me, providing a neat, clean look. Like most people, I went through a period of experimentation, looking for a product which fulfilled all of my needs, and in so doing I discovered two very important don'ts: Don't be swayed by fragrance, and don't be influenced by the amount of lather a shampoo can generate. Neither necessarily makes a shampoo better or

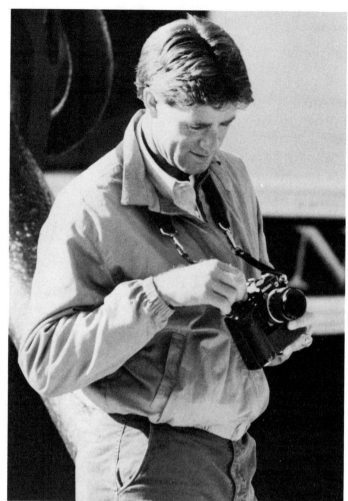

worse. What is important is a product which rids the hair of dirt without robbing it of too much of its natural oil.

The frequency of shampooing really depends on the needs of your hair.

The frequency of shampooing depends on the needs of your hair. I know people who have enough natural oils to feel comfortable shampooing every other day, regardless of their level of physical activity, simply because they feel their scalp will look cleaner and neater. A by-product of this is, of course, that even past age fifty there are

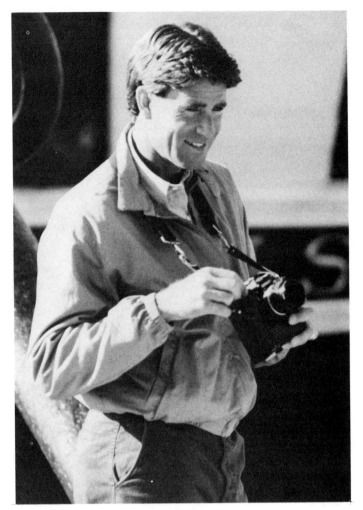

(3) I rinse thoroughly because shampoo can leave a dulling residue on the hair that also can clog the pores.

(4) I repeat the process to further cleanse my hair and scalp and rid it of all residue from the first shampoo.

I also use a separate dressing, VO-5 clear jell, to provide some moisture. When I look in the mirror, I can see if my hair needs a bit of moisture to help it stay in place—and so can you. With the conditioner, I can just fluff my hair a bit and it will keep its proper place.

Of course, much of that is due to the way my hair has been cut and shaped. In other words, my hair fits my head, and here the watchword is simplicity, which is not too difficult now because styles are generally simple and reasonably short.

My hair is parted down the middle, but, like you and everyone else, no doubt, I've gone through many periods of experimentation, gener- ally following the trends of the day. Prior to my current style, I used to wear it parted on the side, but the person who cut my hair said that, given my life as an athlete, it would be a lot easier if my style was such that I could just give it a fluff and a toss and have it fall into place. I'm pretty self- conscious about how my hair looks, so that idea made some sense because, after running around in the outfield for a couple of hours before a game when the temperature was about 95° and the humidity wasn't much lower, I could come away looking like something from outer space.

How are you to know what style may be correct for you?

Begin by taking a good, hard look at yourself in the mirror. Are your ears too prominent? Grow your hair a little long on the sides and comb it over the tops of your ears, or at least allow it to lie next to the ear to minimize the wide open spaces.

Is your forehead too low or too high? If your hairline comes down too far, keep your hair short and brushed back. If it is too high, keep your hair longer, looser and fringed.

What all this equals is giving the impression that your hair fits naturally, and that it naturally frames your face. Often we can delude ourselves into thinking a certain style looks good, or we can be hoodwinked by a so-called specialist who really

no signs of baldness and their manes are hand- some and very becoming. My own experience was that I often would shampoo on a day when I did not pitch simply because I had done so much physical work that I felt I needed a cleaner scalp. Of course, on days I pitched, a post-game shampoo was taken for granted.

In so doing, I also found that there is a proper method to gain the most benefits from shampoo- ing. Here's the regimen which I follow:

(1) Before I get into the shower, I brush my hair vigorously to loosen oil and dirt.

(2) Once in the shower, I wet my hair thoroughly with warm—not hot—water so as not to "shock" the scalp. Then I apply about a tablespoon's worth of shampoo onto the palm of my hand and gently massage it into my scalp.

doesn't know too much. The opinion of your wife or girlfriend isn't always bad because they see you in many different poses and are aware of what makes you look best. Take their opinion, add it to your own and then tell the person who cuts your hair just what you want.

One of the best pieces of advice I ever received was from an art director who worked on some ads I did for Jockey. "Don't get your hair cut too short," he told me. "We think it looks better long." I got the message.

Okay, once you know what you want, how and when do you go about getting it ... it being a haircut? We are, for the moment, not discussing hair styling or permanents. My haircut schedule is geared to my work. If I'm going to pose for Jockey ads, then I try to get a haircut about ten days beforehand. If I'm on a normal routine, then I go every two or three weeks. A good haircut will still look fine after a week, and perhaps will not begin to show increased length for another four or five days.

Actually, when I was playing for the Orioles, getting my hair cut was sometimes a bit of a problem, particularly during spring training. In Florida, I never could get anyone to cut it as I wished, so I'd go six weeks without a haircut. I look at some of the pictures taken of me on opening day and I look like a shaggy dog.

Now I have no problems as long as I can get home within two or three weeks of my last cut, because I have one person who does the job all the time. I found her through a former teammate, Don Stanhouse, a pitcher who had the most unruly head of hair I'd ever seen. She made him look good, and I said if she can make his hair look good, then she should do okay with mine, too.

The first time I went looking for her, she was out of town, so I went to someone else. The result of that venture was having to have my hair cut twice within one week because the first cut just did not work for me. Not work? When he finished, it looked as if *I* had done the work. Later that week the girl Stanhouse used was back in her shop and she took one look at me and said, "Who gave you the zigzag cut?" We talked over what I didn't like and she did a pretty good reclamation job.

I always looked on this exercise as I did my

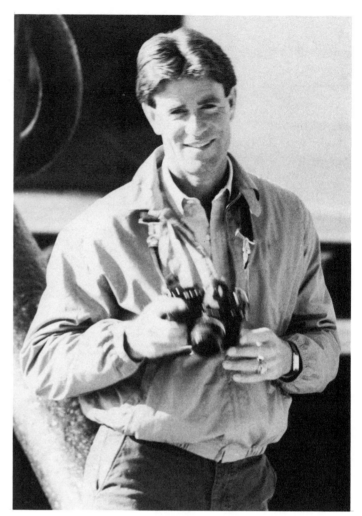

pitching—I prided myself on being a consistent pitcher and all I wanted was someone who would give me, on each visit, the same kind of haircut; someone I could have confidence in every time I sat down and let her go to work. If you can find someone like that, then you are pretty certain to find that correct hair frame.

What about "styling?"

That is individual taste. I don't style mine because I don't want my hair blown, curled, and heated; it can be stretched under those conditions. My personal taste is for a hair style that I can shake with a towel after it dries, add some VO-5 and then just comb back so it will fall into place. That's the case now and it means I don't have to stand in front of a mirror for a long time grooming it.

Then there is the "permanent" look.

I guess I was as surprised as everyone else when my old manager Earl Weaver popped up on television in his first season with ABC with a head of curls. It may have been Earl's way of bridging the gap between his baseball life and his new career, but it didn't last long. He's back with straight hair, cemented down with plenty of hair spray. I told him I'd be afraid to touch his hair for fear I might hurt my hand. Hair spray is not for me because it makes my hair too stiff.

Seriously, if you think you will look good with a permanent, then you should seek the proper advice and go for it if the reasons are sound. I once thought about getting one because it is very easy to care for, but then I heard a couple of horror stories which backed me off. While working on a spread for *Town and Country,* I had met a photographer's assistant who literally had no hair. He told me he had gotten a perm and most of it wound up on his pillow. Evidently it was treated wrong and he hadn't used the proper conditioner. Something as different-looking as a permanent demands the coolest possible judgement, and you must envision how you will look. A lot of people simply don't look good with curly hair.

A stylist still pushes me to get one and I told her that if you really want to curl my hair, let's do it without using the solutions so I can see how it looks before getting too far committed for something that will last three or four months. That's as far as the idea has gone—and will ever go, I imagine.

But, again, don't let me dissuade you if you ardently want a perm. Just be sure you have covered all the bases I've described.

Of course, the flip side of all of this is the guy who may be losing his hair or already has lost most of it. I am totally sensitive to his feelings because I know how much I value my healthy crop, and I can imagine my feelings if it should begin to disappear.

I've known scores of young athletes, including many former teammates, who've fought the problem, and really there was little they could do but learn to cope, or get some expert advice on how to compensate. Sometimes the coping becomes a bit tough when there are insensitive people around, but you can do a lot to help yourself in such situations.

Strive for naturalness.

Strive for naturalness and don't try to get too much from what you have, because that way you will just make yourself look more unnatural. Resolve in your own mind that you're bald or getting there, and so what? Telly Savalas and Yul Brynner became sex symbols without hair.

Of course, there are alternatives such as hair-weaving, transplants, wigs and toupees, but get the very best professional advice before launching into any of those ventures and then be prepared for the reactions which may follow from the sudden change in your appearance.

About ten years ago a friend in Baltimore who owns a restaurant decided to try a hairpiece and he wanted me to look at the final product before he went home to show it to his wife.

It didn't look too bad to me, but as soon as we walked into his house, his wife took one look and said, "You gotta be kidding!"

Naturally, he was taken aback by the less than enthusiastic response and said, "Well, get used to it because what you see now is what you're going to see forever."

That same evening while we were sitting in his living room waiting for his attorney's son, little did we know that the boy had come to the house, looked in the window, saw what he thought was a strange man, and went away believing he had the wrong address.

Things didn't get any better when my friend came down to spring training to visit me. We went to restaurants frequented by Baltimoreans and, as visible as he always had been from his own restaurant business, no one even recognized him.

Gradually through the years he and his hairpiece became as one in the eyes of all, and he updated it and changed it somewhat. Last year, though, I noticed that during the hot afternoons he'd take it off, so I took a few hard looks at him and decided he really didn't look that bad all natural. When he put it back on, I saw that time had taken a toll and it no longer enhanced his appearance.

Finally, he did away with it, and when he returned to his restaurant, people would come up to him and say, "Hey, you lost weight, didn't you?"

"No," he'd say.

"Well, there's something different about you." And he'd just smile and let matters pass on.

I still advise letting yourself be, keeping what hair you have short and leaving it alone. Your face is what people notice first about you.

One final hair topic: beards and moustaches. If your face doesn't need the frame of either, then avoid them. Certainly, a weak chin gains strength from even a short beard, and a moustache can make some faces interesting. But if you simply do it for a "macho" look, it will more likely be a distraction than add anything positive to your appearance. Harmony, naturalness and common sense should be your guides.

Be yourself ... and you won't go wrong.

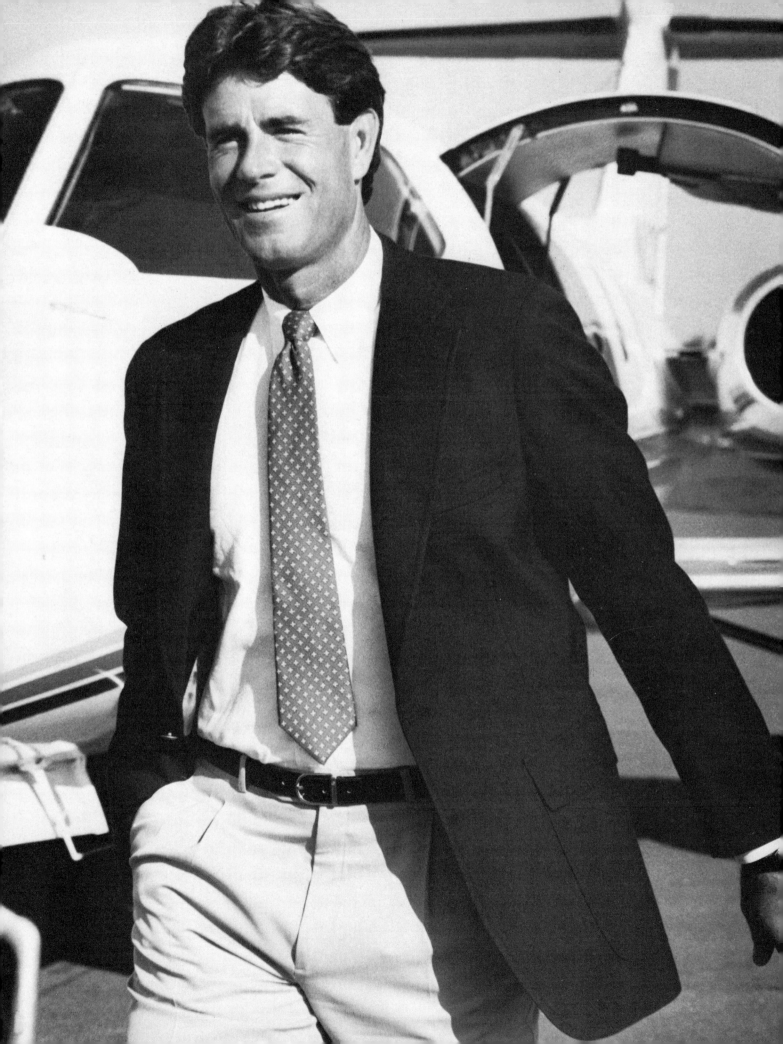

CHAPTER 7

FASHION FIT: SMART DRESSING FOR ALL OCCASIONS

You've heard the old bromide about how "clothes make the man." Well, let me say that they don't always do a complete job, but a man certainly can add the correct finishing touch with the proper use of his wardrobe.

That doesn't mean you must have closets filled with clothes, because it's not the quantity and not always the quality that counts most. It is what you do with what is best for you.

I have had problems all my life getting what I want, when I want it and in the style which will look best. In fact, I really envy those of you who can go into a clothing store, select what you want, have it fitted on the spot and then walk out with your purchase, or else know that within a few days it will be ready and be in your closet within hours. I can't do that because, at six-feet-four-inches, I have a size problem—I'm kind of in-between everything, and buying clothes is sort of an ordeal.

During all my seasons with the Orioles, I was subject to a strict team dress code. The Orioles were one of the few teams in all of professional sports to maintain such a rule after styles became so casual. Until just the last couple of seasons, we had to wear a coat and tie on our road trips at all times—and only ties have been eliminated—which was something that our management copied from those great Yankee teams of the fifties. In fact, during spring training in Miami, for years we had to wear a coat and tie after seven o'clock in the evening. The dress code wasn't always popular, but I found that most of us really wanted to look good, and it really was a pleasure to have someone come up and say, "Gee, who is this group of nice-looking young men? You're so well dressed."

Of course, we didn't always appreciate it and were constantly trying to get the rule changed. I guess everything came apart in this regard when we barnstormed home from spring training with the Yankees a few years back and they wore T-shirts, sandals, jeans, just about anything they

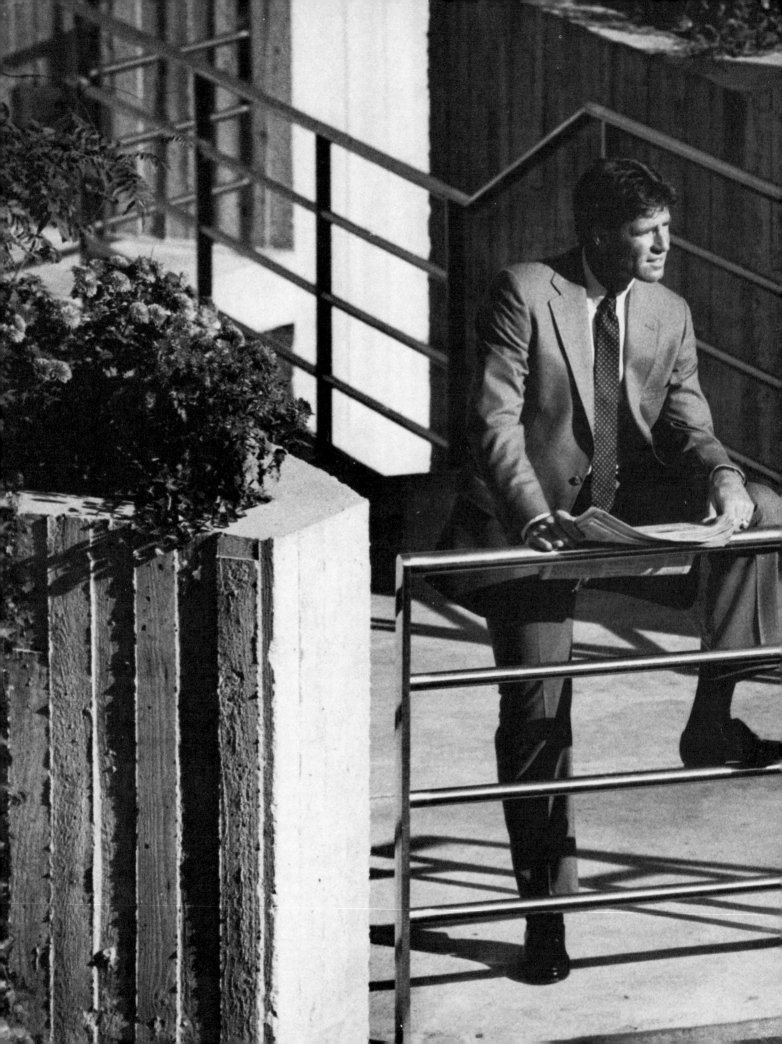

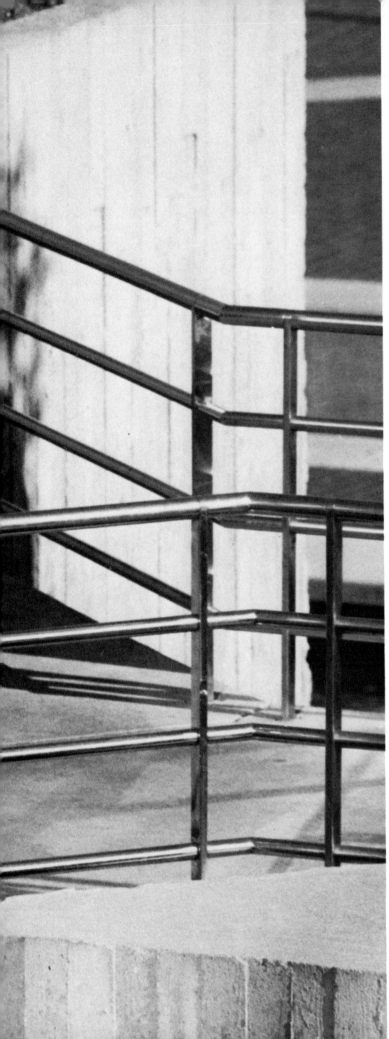

wished. If our management was thinking about amending the rules, it took one look at the Yankees and reconsidered.

Back in 1967, my third season with the Orioles, Hank Bauer then was our manager and turtlenecks came into vogue. Hank was a former Yankee player who grew up in the big leagues with our same dress code, and when I asked about substituting a turtleneck for shirt and tie, he wouldn't budge.

"Oh, no," he said, "you guys will wind up wearing those mock turtle shirts."

"Well," I pressed on, "why not make a rule that there'll be no mock turtles, just turtlenecks. If you're worried about wearing mock turtles or just turtlenecks, just eliminate one or the other."

Somehow, my logic escaped him and we stayed with coats and ties—and there were no deviations from the rule, even in the seventies when styles became more casual. Reggie Jackson discovered that fact during his only season with us in 1976. Reggie said, "I don't own a tie." "We assume you make enough money, so why don't you buy one?" our manager, Earl Weaver, replied.

Yet when we began our first road trip, Reggie showed up not wearing a tie and Earl told him, "You can't get on the plane."

One of the other guys had brought a tie for him, though really the players were looking forward to this confrontation between our newest star and Earl because they wanted the rule changed. So Reggie wore the tie, but when we landed and were about to board our bus for the hotel, it was already in his pocket. Of course, to get on the bus, the tie rule still was in effect, so Earl called him over in the airport and said, "You're going to have to take a cab unless you put on your tie."

Reggie just looked at him. "What do you mean? I'm wearing a $395 Raphael jacket, $125 Gucci loafers, $85 gabardine slacks; I have a Gucci belt, a Gucci shirt, my El Presidente Rolex watch," and he went on and on, like he had priced everything he wore. To no avail—he put on the tie.

The next day when we boarded our bus to go to the ballpark, Tony Muser, one of our utility infielders, had a tag on his jacket that read,

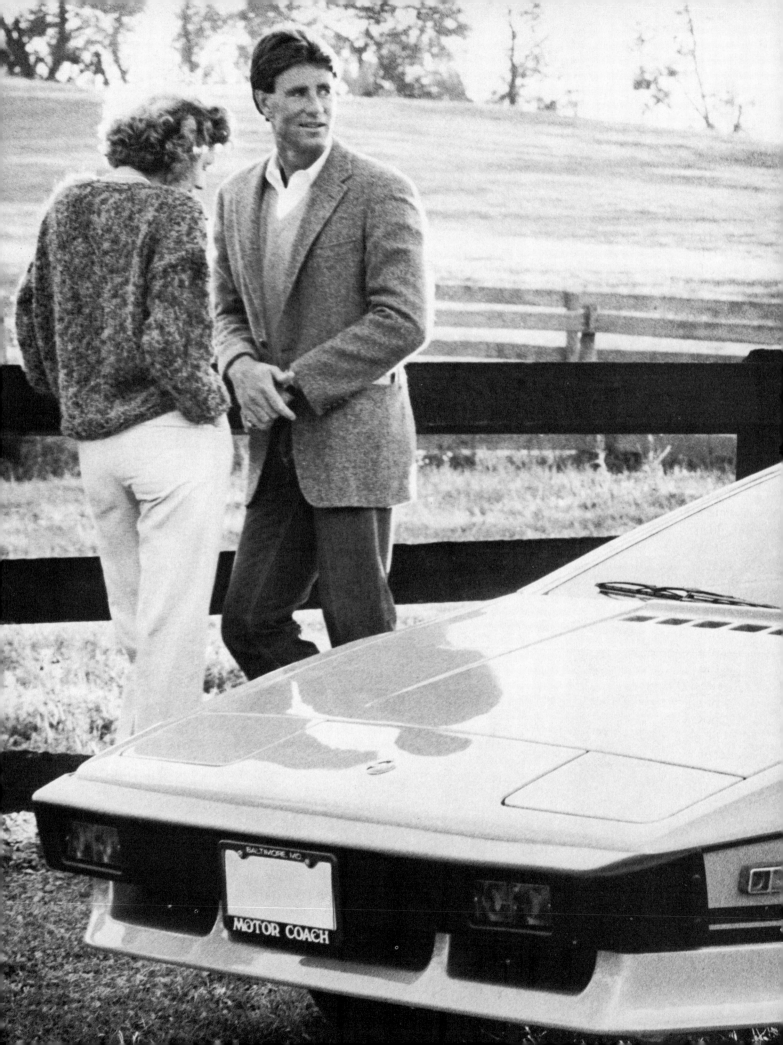

"$29.95" ... one on his shirt that said "$9.95" ... a price tag on everything he wore. Everyone appreciated the humor except Reggie, but the point was well taken. Yet I sympathized with Jackson a little because he was immaculately dressed even if he didn't conform to the rules by wearing a tie. He thought he looked good, and I certainly couldn't disagree.

In looking back, I didn't always like our dress code, but I do believe that it made us care how we looked and helped us to take a little pride in our appearance. We had players like Reggie, Frank Robinson and Lee May who were always well dressed, regardless of where we went. That was just their way, and you couldn't help but learn something from that.

Certainly, as young men, ballplayers are not immune to trends and styles and usually have enough money to go after them. There are few businesses where the employees dress and undress together, and I first saw the evolution of new styles in the colored underwear which the players began wearing almost a decade ago—and I don't say that simply to plug my affiliation with Jockey. Then came blow dryers after showers—heck, when they build new stadiums or renovate old ones, architects will have to include electrical outlets in all of the lockers so players can plug in their dryers, to say nothing of the other appliances which many now carry around.

So you can't be on a major-league ball club without being aware of new trends and styles. Because I have been around the horn a few times on the subject, I have come to appreciate just what it takes to achieve the correct look, which is made up of such elements as fit, style, selection and purpose. We'll look at all of them as we seek to cover what by now should be a well-conditioned and properly coiffed and clean body.

The first commandment is that clothing need not be expensive or complicated.

The first commandment is that clothing need not be expensive or complicated. A good wardrobe isn't necessarily huge, because it is possible to look your best when the clothes you wear for any occasion mesh to produce a single and harmonious impression. I go right back to a theme that has pretty much run through this book: simplicity and doing what best suits you.

Begin by taking a good look at yourself in a full-length mirror and determining just what kind of body frame you must cover. Believe it or not, you come in one of three sizes—endomorph, ectomorph, or mesomorph, meaning that you are:

(1) Endomorph: short, 5'7" or less, tending toward stockiness.

(2) Mesomorph: naturally proportioned, neither too wide nor too narrow. Usually 5'8" to 6'2".

(3) Ectomorph: tall, 6'3" or more, and long-limbed. That's me.

What does all of that mean in terms of clothing selection? Here are some general pointers about what kind of fit, fabrics and colors to choose for your wardrobe:

(1) *Endomorph:* If you are shorter than you'd like to appear, or just plain short, choose smooth fabrics; textured, nubby clothing will make you appear wider and squarer. Wear matching or closely related colors so as not to distract the eye with too great a color contrast. Remember, wildly different colors emphasize the horizontal rather than the vertical. Wear unpleated trousers, which give a simple rather than fussy effect. Choose pants with a relatively high waist and narrow belts. Keep your shirt collars narrow rather than wide. Wear medium-toned clothes. Stay away from those which are too light or too dark.

(2) *Mesomorph:* You can wear just about anything within traditional stylistic parameters. No problem when you walk into a clothing store. Congratulations!

(3) *Ectomorph:* Choose pleated pants, which will make your legs seem wider. If possible, wear flap pockets for added visual interest that distracts from your vertical look. Wear textured cloth such as wools or tweeds which give a wider effect, and don't be afraid of plaids. Keep your jacket shoulders natural and rounded. Wear wider trousers and stick to darker colors or a small overall design, preferably

in unshiny cloth. The texture of your clothing should be "matte."

If you still are overweight and don't wish to wait for our exercise and nutrition program to take full effect, the last part of the ectomorph look—natural, rounded-shouldered jackets, wider trousers of dark colors and unshiny cloth—can serve as good camouflage until the real you has emerged.

Now a word of understanding and encouragement to you ectomorphs—and anyone else who, like me, needs an in-between size that begs proper fitting. I'm between a long and an extra long, and if you ever picked up a fashion magazine such as *Gentleman's Quarterly* and saw something that you liked, then you know it is almost impossible to purchase it off the rack.

Okay, so perhaps we can afford to find a tailor who will make what we want, but the problem here is that it may take two or three months before it is finished, so you lose all the enthusiasm of getting something you like at the moment you see it. I've even had trouble buying socks, which may sound like a simple item, but if you don't go to a tall or big men's store and buy over-the-calf socks which are made for men 6'4" and over, then those which you may purchase keep falling down. Nothing is more uncomfortable than wearing socks which are supposed to be over the calf and have them constantly at midcalf or coming down around your ankles.

Suits are another problem. I used to weigh 210 pounds—I'm now at 190—and took a size 44 suit jacket, almost a size 46, but my waist was 34 or 35. But the pants with a suit jacket that size were 38 or 39, so I had to have them recut, and the back pockets ended up looking like Siamese twins.

While I was working on the pilot show for a proposed TV series recently, the producers asked for my clothing size. Thinking they were going to purchase clothes off the rack, I simply said, "Extra long." Later I found out they'd had the clothes specially made, and if I had known that beforehand, I could have told them to make my jacket 34 inches long—a long is 33 inches and an extra long is 35, which is why I'm in between. So I wound up wearing a coat 35 inches long, which

didn't look too bad but it really missed the correct proportions.

I pay close attention to how my clothes fit.

However difficult, I pay close attention to how my clothes fit even though I sometimes settle for a 35-inch coat rather than one that is 34 inches. Ever since I was a kid, I've been a bit paranoid about having my trousers too short, my jacket hiking up in the back and my shoes too small.

What fed that fear stemmed from contracting a case of lead poisoning in my left arm from an errant pencil when I was in seventh grade. I had penicillin shots to get rid of the poisoning, but as I continued to grow I noticed trouble with my heels to the point of having a problem putting on my shoes. Since I was playing year-round sports at the time, my parents took me to a foot specialist and after he examined my feet, he said, "The way your feet are built you should be wearing size-fifteen shoes, but because of the lead poisoning, your toes apparently didn't grow as long as they should. What you have is a foot frame that probably is size fifteen and an actual foot size for a fourteen shoe."

Of course, as a kid I feared that the company which made Bostonian shoes, the only ones that fit my size-14 feet, would cease production and leave me, at worst, barefoot forever or, at best, with a tattered pair of shoes which might have to last from age twelve until the day I died. Silly? Of course, but it left an impression that hasn't diminished as I continue to seek proper size and fit.

Of course, tall people such as myself can go into a tall men's shop now, but there weren't any when I was growing up. If I do buy off the rack, it will often be a European brand or something by Perry Ellis or Ralph Lauren, who make oversize clothes. If I buy a Lauren rugby shirt, the sleeves are going to be too long, but to me that's almost refreshing.

Shirts with sleeves too long don't sound too

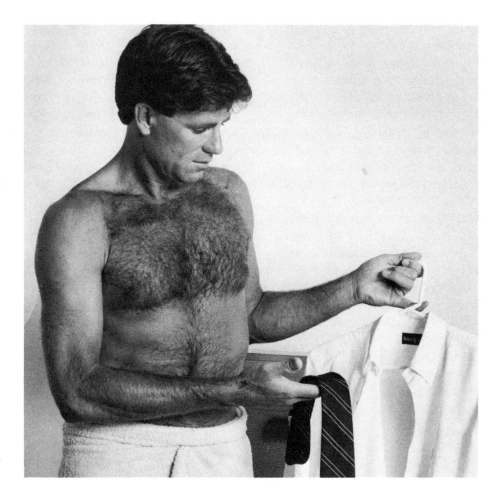

stylish, you say, and perhaps you are correct, but I have never been hung up on what is "stylish" because that can be so fleeting, or else not really Jim Palmer. I'm basically a very conservative person in my outlook, and my clothes naturally reflect this part of my personality.

For instance, I can't ever see myself in the Italian look or some of the other looks you find in *Gentleman's Quarterly* because I would never even be able to try them on. And if I could, the question would be: Am I comfortable wearing them? I have a $3,500 Russian raccoon coat that my former wife thought I would look good in. Now, I'm allergic to cats and I think I'm allergic to that wonderful jacket. That's too bad because it's beautiful, it's very warm, but still, being a somewhat shy person, I don't like to draw attention to myself with such an unusual piece of clothing. If anything, I probably try to

downplay who I am and therefore I just dress very conservatively.

And for a few other reasons, too. First, it is easy to find conservative clothes; second, traditional clothes last longer; and third, it is very hard for me to buy anything other than traditional clothes.

Dress as you really are; to feel comfortable as you, the person.

So the key bit of advice here is to dress as you really are; to feel comfortable as you, the person, must be; and don't get caught up in styles just for the sake of styles. Be yourself. You'll look better and you'll feel better.

Okay, you say, then what should I wear?

The key here is to strive for a natural overall look. Clothing is one area where you can, through variety and what appeals to you, make a very personal statement about yourself, your personality and your taste. If you choose properly, I believe you'll automatically boost your self-confidence.

The first step, after knowing your body type, is to get your clothes fitted to its contours. I strongly recommend that you go to a men's store that will alter your clothes as well as fit your natural body line. Have an expert adjust your clothing so that it works with your body type and body movement, not against it. You'll quickly learn to feel what fits right, and eventually you'll be able to choose off-the-rack yourself, provided you're not an in-betweener like me.

Now, what to purchase?

I'm a big believer in the so-called "classics"—styles which have withstood years of change and which you can build your wardrobe around. You can wear them for every occasion without fearing you are being over- or underdressed. Let's break this down into your requirements for business—which really means semiformal occasions when custom dictates wearing a jacket and tie—and for sports and leisure occasions.

For the *Semiformal Occasions:*

1 navy-blue suit. Avoid black, which either means you're in mourning or you're wearing a tux.

1 gray suit

1 tan suit (but not too light a tan)

1 navy-blue blazer

1 or 2 pairs of gray flannel trousers

Ties:

Maroon, navy blue, conservative stripe, polka dot. Vary these a bit. Sometimes a brightly colored tie can give just the right casual impression. And if you're short—an endomorph, remember?—brightening the top of your frame will draw the eye upward.

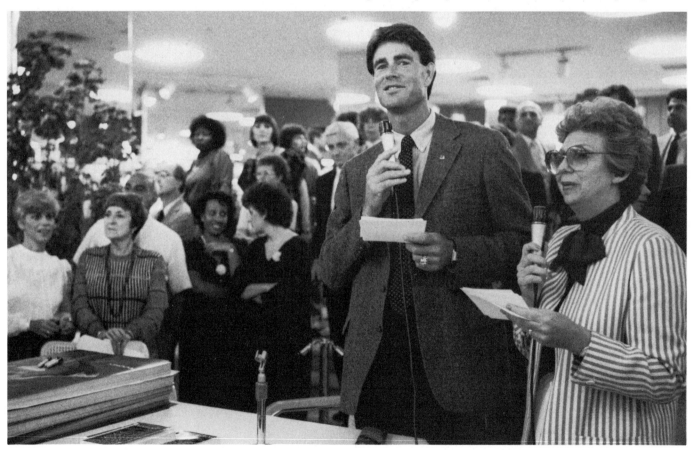

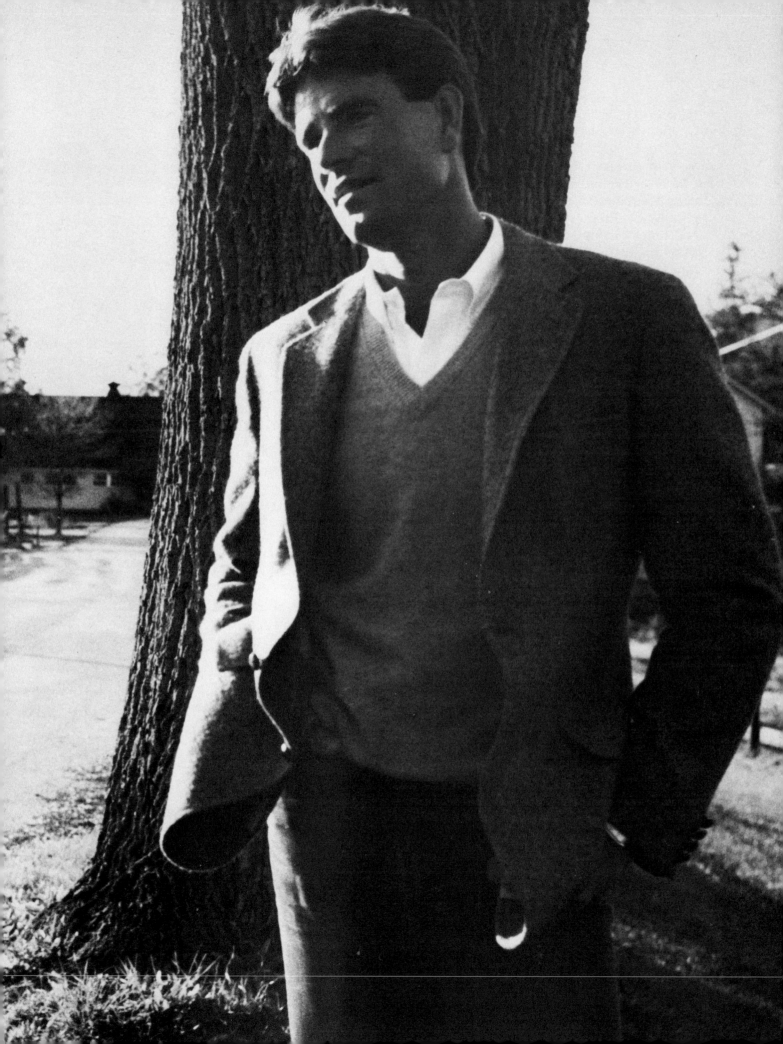

Socks:

2 pairs dark blue, 2 pairs gray, 1 pair dark brown. I know people who have a drawer filled with all dark blue or all black socks so that when socks begin to disappear (washing machines seem to have an insatiable hunger for one sock!) they can sooner or later match a pair. Your sock color should relate to but not necessarily match the color of your tie. And I prefer the full calf-length socks. Short socks showing hairy bare legs somehow take away from the overall picture.

Shoes:

Like suits, these are investments, so strive for quality and they'll last longer and look better. 2 pairs black, 1 tie shoe, 1 pull-on loafer; 1 pair brown, either tie or pull-on.

Shirts:

2 white, 2 light blue, 2 or 3 others at your discretion; and of course you can increase this number proportionately if it is a long time between laundries. But stick to light pastels or lightly patterned types.

Now for some general guidelines once you've accumulated this wardrobe:

(1) Take care of your clothes, meaning hang them on the appropriate hangers. Draping them over chairs or nudged on hooks distorts their shape; and leaving them on the floor all but destroys it and simply adds to your pressing and dry-cleaning bills.

(2) Keep fabrics natural, preferably cotton and wool or a mixture of natural and polyester, with more natural than synthetic, because clothes look better when they're made of natural fibers and they breathe better, which means you'll be more comfortable.

For *Sports and Leisure Wear* your personal taste can have a freer reign, and what I will suggest can be used only as a general guide:

Sweaters:

A variety of colors, but stick with natural fibers. A variety of sweaters, both long-sleeved and vest style, worn under a sports jacket or alone, can make your wardrobe seem greater than it is.

Sports jackets:

1 "earth"-colored tweed jacket, 1 blazer, more casual and a different color than your navy-blue classic, 1 plaid or lighter-colored jacket, something that truly appeals to you.

Trousers:

2 or 3 pairs of jeans, and don't be afraid to wear them with a tweed jacket for casual occasions, 1 pair of chinos but in a muted color, 1 or 2 pairs of cords, tan and whatever other color you prefer.

Casual Shirts:

Cotton knit short-sleeved, flannel, plaids. The key is variety, so choose from 4 to 10 or even more, in different colors.

There is one other area regarding your clothes.

Certainly the sports-and-leisure group are suitable for the ever-increasing travel which all of us are required to do. As I noted, we had a dress code on the Orioles, but the suit jacket and tie routine didn't end with our traveling as a group. Since we often stayed in one city three or four days, the players made good use of coat and tie, and even suits, during our road trips.

When I travel for business, I wear something casual, perhaps a blazer with a pair of slacks and maybe just a button-down shirt. I know I'm easily recognized and that my work necessarily casts a certain image, so I can't go around looking shabby. It just isn't my style to go out in public looking that way.

I certainly consider it well within normal bounds of neatness to wear docksiders and a pair of pressed khaki slacks and a sports or waist-length jacket on a plane or to a casual social event, because they fit that particular occasion. But if I am going to a business meeting or an important social affair where I must wear a tie, then I definitely will wear regular shoes, gabardine slacks and a good blazer or sports jacket, or perhaps solve all problems by wearing a suit.

And what do I wear underneath all of this?

Well, there is this underwear company that manufactures a dynamite line of briefs. Perhaps you've heard me mention it....

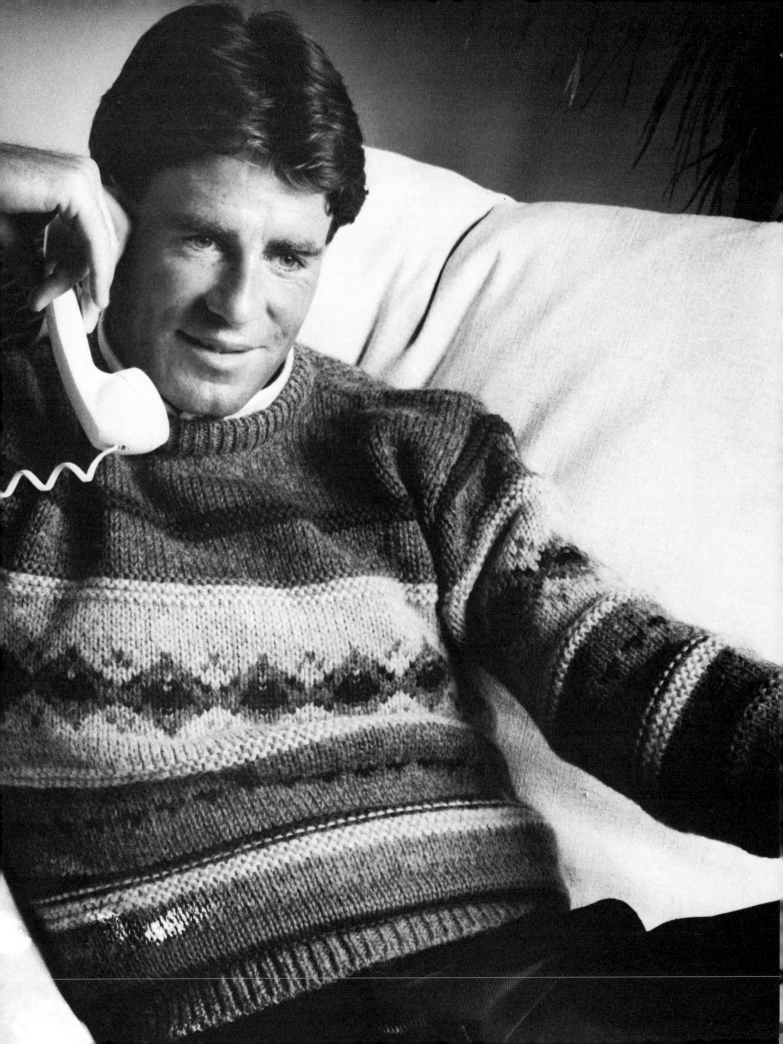

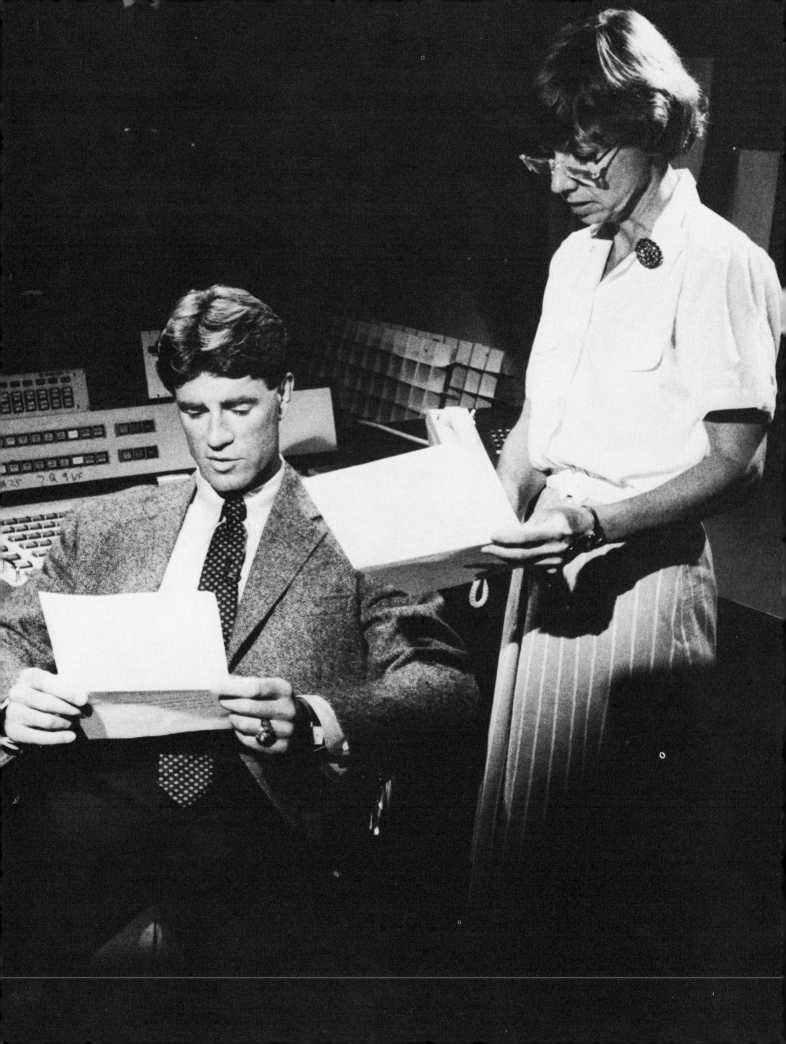

CHAPTER 8

BOTTOM OF THE NINTH; BASES LOADED, TWO OUTS AND FULL COUNT... OR HOW TO HANDLE STRESS

By this time I hope that I've given you some very good ideas on how to improve your life and lifestyle, but, honestly, there is more to that subject than just physical exercise and making yourself look good. There is a subject of living—let's call it *coping*—where you must find a way to be successful in what you do, particularly in your professional life.

Some call it stress management, and my quick solution for managing stress was always to pitch a three-hit shutout. You can't lose, and most likely you'll win.

But shutouts often were elusive targets in baseball just as they are in life. Yet every time I walked to the mound to pitch, I faced the problem of stress, and it came in many different flavors— regular season, all-star game, league championship and World Series. Sometimes I pitched those three-hit shutouts, often I didn't, but still I had to cope because I was expected to win almost every time I

worked, and, regardless of what my career records say, it never was really easy.

But then, I don't believe that life—yours or mine—is always meant to be easy or stress-free.

Perhaps a few of my own insights and experiences may make that life's path a little smoother. I certainly am not a snake-oil salesman for instant pop psychology or a pulpit bully who is about to preach fire and brimstone. But laying down some of my experiences—good and bad— and how I've coped with them may find a responsive chord and give you some ideas on how to master your own problems and manage your daily affairs.

To begin, some thoughts about the life of an athlete, and how it mirrors, in many ways, life in the "real world." Playing professional sports and whatever you do in that "real world" have one common ground: Produce or be gone. I know that with all of the attention given to the huge salaries paid to some athletes, the common perception is that they really don't work for a living, and that they have no real idea of what "ordinary" people must face every day.

Athletes and coaches either pass or fail every time they are on the field.

Some of that may be true because there is no doubt that professional athletes are amply compensated in relation to what 99 percent of the population receives, and that they do exist in a sort of special world where adulation and recognition prevail. There is no doubt, too, that many athletes really do lose contact with the struggles which so many people undergo in their daily lives, and often are unprepared themselves for entry into this world. The smart ones look ahead to the time when the game-playing stops for them and they take advantage of all that is offered until that time comes.

But there also is a similarity that very much mirrors the life which people like yourself must endure, and which, quite honestly, seems to be overlooked when all of the gold and glory aspects of pro sports are discussed.

Simply stated, athletes and coaches must either pass or fail every time they are on the field, be it almost daily during the baseball season, thrice weekly during the hockey or basketball season, or weekly during football season. My friends in the business world, many just like you, I'm sure, may work on a project that must be completed over a period of months before a verdict of success or failure can be rendered. A starting pitcher walks to the mound every four days and he either wins or he doesn't; a football coach has only a week to prepare several dozen players for the literally hundreds of things which can confront his team, and either he and his team succeed or they don't.

The point here is that athletes and coaches, money and glory aside, work under very stressful conditions and, depending upon the sport, often under extreme physical and emotional circum-

stances as well. In the two or three hours in which they compete, there is no time for lengthy meetings and consultations, and they can't wait for better market conditions.

All professional athletes must learn from the very first day how to work within this pressurized environment, with its slings and arrows providing myriads of distractions as well as excuses and reasons to fail. Performance is all that matters; and winning performance is all that counts.

And it is not just the players who are affected. Many of you are probably in some management capacity, or soon will be, where you must get the most from those in your charge under competitive market conditions, with your opposite in the competing firm facing the same situations and problems. Neither of you is any different from the manager or coach who must work with anywhere from a dozen to 100 players and extract from them the same kind of winning performance against his opposite number.

The key to reducing this pressure is preparation.

Pure and simple, that is stress, or pressure. The key to lessening this pressure is preparation, which really is the basic philosophy of this book. If you want to look good and be fit, then you must prepare for those results by doing what we have laid out.

If you are prepared, then you will be confident, and confidence is the breeding ground for success. Simply stated, that means do your homework—get yourself ready so that when you face a decision or a crisis you will have all the facts at hand, you will have already explored the options; and you will know the probable consequences of anything you may do.

In a baseball sense, I equate that to a pitcher who prepares for his starting assignments by doing more than just throwing or strengthening his arm. He does his daily running; on the bench during the games, he pays attention to how the opposition's hitters react to certain pitches and what they

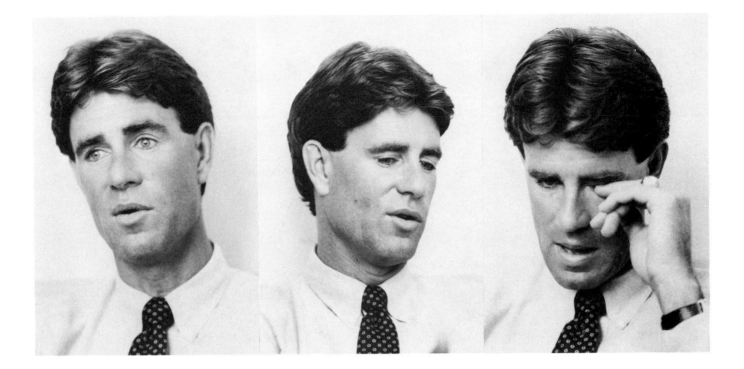

do in certain situations; he listens to his pitching coach, and if he's a young pitcher just getting started, he talks as much as possible to the veteran players.

When I started with the Orioles, I used to sit in our bullpen and listen to veterans like Dick Hall, Stu Miller and Harvey Haddix, and then I had a marvelous teacher in my first roommate, Robin Roberts, who now is in the Hall of Fame. The club put us together because I was young and they felt I could be successful. Robby and I talked a lot about pitching, particularly about what he did when he was a young pitcher, and he convinced me that the best pitch in baseball is a good fastball. That was my pitch then and it stayed my best pitch for most of my career because I was totally confident of its success.

In fact, throughout my career, when I had a 3–2 count on a batter, I never once threw a curve ball because I wasn't as confident of my ability to get that pitch over the plate. I tried to do what I did best, which meant I recognized my limitations and attempted to reduce them to the minimum. That principle was drummed home by every pitching instructor in the Orioles organization—

throw the ball over the plate, and in a crucial part of the game, use your best pitches and pitch within your capabilities.

We always tried to expand those capabilities with our work before each start so that in a game we had more going for us. What it came down to was not throwing your third or fourth best pitch and having it beat you in a certain situation. I recall watching Mike Flanagan lose to the Kansas City Royals on television a few years ago when Amos Otis hit his slider for a home run.

"The wasn't the right pitch to throw in that situation," I told Mike the next time I saw him.

"Why?" he asked me, obviously very insulted.

"Is that your first, second, third or fourth best pitch?" I replied.

Mike just nodded. It certainly wasn't his best. Try to succeed with your best, if at all possible.

I guess this same idea came to my mind during a game against the Texas Rangers in 1973 when I had retired the first twenty-five batters, meaning I was just two outs—two batters—away from pitching a perfect game. Now, I had already thrown a no-hitter six years before, so the

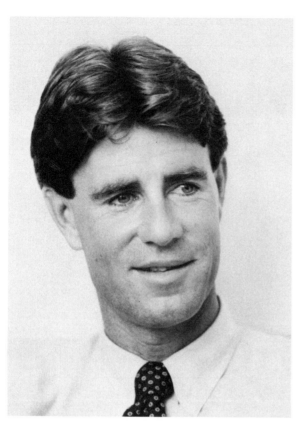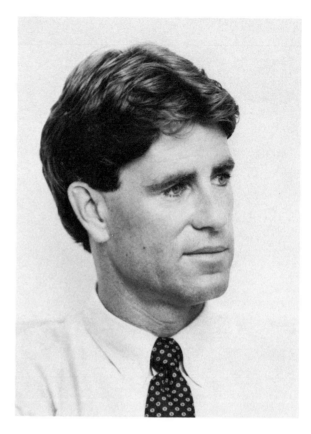

perfectionist in me said, "Why not be perfect this time?"

I got behind 2–0 to the twenty-sixth batter and I was faced with two options: Either work around the guy and perhaps walk him, spoiling my perfect game but still giving me a shot at a no-hitter; or go for the perfect game by giving him a ball to hit and hoping it would go to someone. I always thought in terms of perfection, so I said, "Okay, go ahead and hit it," and he did, right through the middle for a single. I lost the no-hitter perfect game and ultimately wound up with a two-hit shutout. But I felt more comfortable striving for perfection.

A great dividend from preparation is greater concentration.

Looking back at my career, I lost 152 games—that's almost an entire season (162 games)—but rarely was I unprepared to pitch, which is partly why I also won 268. The bottom line in preparation for me—and for you, too—is that when you go out and do your job, even if you don't succeed, you know you prepared yourself as well as possible and maybe this time somebody was just a little better. A great dividend from preparation is greater concentration. One of the questions I'm always asked was how did I concentrate in front of thousands of screaming people. I always said that my best games were the ones where there was a direct line between the catcher and myself and I never noticed anything that was happening around me. It also was obvious when that wasn't happening. During our first game after the 1978 All-Star game, when my pitch selection and location were sloppy, Doug DeCinces, our third baseman, walked over to the mound and said, "Where are you tonight?"

"I don't know, but it's certainly not here," I told him—and I wasn't, at least not mentally.

I never had any special routine to get me into that kind of mind-set, but we had a couple of

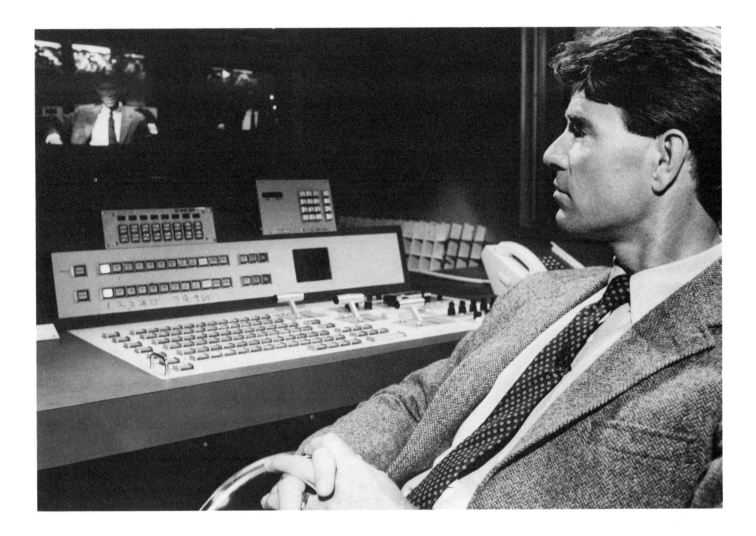

pitchers who used to sit alone in the shower room, without the water running, trying to meditate and get themselves mentally ready for the game. We had another who went into a closet and closed the door to do his meditation. Jim Hardin, who was with us in the late sixties and early seventies, learned self-hypnosis when he played winter ball in Puerto Rico. He had programmed his mind to respond to the word "jam" to trigger his concentration effort. Earl Weaver brought a guy in from Chicago and had him try hypnosis on me a couple of times during a season, but it never really worked. What he tried to do was to get me to relax and get my mind tuned into my body and build up self-confidence that way.

But, all the special techniques aside, nothing takes the place of being prepared, and you can understand, I believe, how it can lessen the

pressure on yourself. Do it often enough and it becomes second nature, and works for anything you might be involved in.

A case in point:

A couple of years ago I was invited to appear on the David Letterman show, which follows the Carson show late at night. I always appreciated David's humor, but I knew that he could really do a job on you. Fortunately, the night before the show, I was at a sports banquet and mentioned my appearance to Tug McGraw, the Phillies' fine relief pitcher.

"I know he's going to work me over about my underwear modeling," I said to Tug. "What can I do other than hope he'll show a little mercy to a fraternity brother?"

"I know what you mean," Tug replied. "I was on his show and the only thing to do is to keep talking and don't let him get a word in edgewise. That's your only hope."

So I did, and when it ended, we had had a tremendous time and my fears never were realized. But if I hadn't taken some pains to find out how to cope with David, then I probably would have become a well-dressed dartboard for his humor.

I still get nervous when I have to give a speech, but I try to prepare so that I won't make a fool of myself. In fact, I get just as nervous doing that as I did pitching, and I went to the mound with the same apprehension in the last game I ever pitched as I did in the first one.

I've carried this same philosophy into my broadcasting work, and with the other business interests in which I am becoming involved. I feel the same uneasiness that I did when I pitched—not that this is bad because I never want to feel so comfortable that I will take anything for granted. I could go into a broadcasting booth and wing it for the entire game, but I've seen that the best broadcasters—like the best pitchers—are the best-prepared craftsmen. When I have prepared for a job, the stress and anxiety are reduced, and that alone is worth the effort.

Of course, I realize that there can be outside forces which also can add stress. I had Earl Weaver to contend with for most of my major-league career and I think our differences are well known by now. Looking back, I always felt that Earl and I were too much alike to get along—both of us wanted to win so badly, that neither of us would tolerate any excuses for it not happening, him with me, and me with him.

I've always wondered what it would have been like to have played for another manager.

Still, I've always wondered what it would have been like to play for another manager. Earl never once shook my hand after I had won a game—and I won over two hundred for him—because his philosophy was that if I shake your hand when you win, what do I do when you lose?

So he preferred to be a one-way guy—totally indifferent in a personal sense all the time. Yet I have seen Sparky Anderson of the Tigers kibbitz and congratulate his pitchers, and Ralph Houk always was the first guy out of the dugout after his guy had won a game.

The only time I ever heard what amounted to a "thank you" from Earl came two days after he stopped managing, when we were broadcasting the American League playoffs for ABC. This was Earl's first exposure as a TV analyst and I knew the network had put us together hoping that we might strike a few sparks from our well-publicized feud.

But I wasn't thinking about that because I still was so bitterly disappointed at having lost the final game of the 1982 season against Milwaukee that prevented us from winning the division title. At one point in the telecast I simply vented my disappointment over the air, and was genuinely surprised—and pleased—when Earl said, "Jimmy, you have nothing to be ashamed of. You gave it your best shot and that's all you could have done."

I protested further, but he waved me off, telling me not to worry about it. I know he was as disappointed as I—probably more so because it was his final game and he wanted nothing more than to end with a World Series victory, which of course vanished in that loss.

If you are in a managerial position, don't be afraid to say "Thanks" or "Well done." All of us need this, regardless of our achievements. More often than not, you will find the dividends being repaid in harder work, greater loyalty and a fierce pride that no amount of money can purchase. Competitive athletics and business are no different in this respect, because people, with all of their emotions, are involved and ultimately it is people who will determine success.

I believe this is particularly true for a person who always is expected to succeed. You may be one of those; you may have one in your charge. I always felt that great expectations were placed on me because of my talent and performance, and I accepted it. Still, I also felt that if I pitched 290 innings a season, Earl would have wanted 300.

In a sense, that was a back-handed compliment because he felt I was the best pitcher he had and he never wanted me to come out of a game. And believe me, there were times late in games when I wanted to come out because I had nothing left. Sometimes he refused to lift me. "You won Cy Young Awards finishing games, and if I take you out, I've got nobody out there [in the bullpen] who can do the job better," he'd say.

That, of course, wasn't true, because our bullpen was always pretty strong, but I stayed in and sometimes I got pounded. Yet there also were occasions when I'd get in a jam because a couple of our outfielders collided on a surefire out and suddenly runners were in scoring position with none out.

Out Earl would come, and I'd be thinking, "What now?"

Out Earl would come, and I'd be thinking, "What now?"

"Don't worry about it," he'd sometimes say. "You can't win by yourself."

Attitudes such as this touch on a leadership or managerial quality. They can inspire confidence and send a person to greater heights. At the same time, there also are qualities needed to help subordinates get over a failed situation. Early in my Orioles career we had a pitching coach who always had his arm around the winning pitcher, but the loser was a bad guy. When people are successful, they don't need a pat on the fanny. It's when they are failing and things are going badly that they need someone to give them some kind of consolation.

In a success-oriented business such as base-ball—and perhaps in your business as well—the success of every participant ultimately determines the success of the manager. Often those who fail are left to cope with their own problems—and that is wrong. A person's career can often be saved with a little caring.

The biggest turnabout in my career came under such conditions. In 1968, after flopping around the Orioles' minor-league system for nearly

two seasons trying to recover from a series of ailments and get my pitching in order, I finished the year in the Instructional League. In my final game there, it was like batting practice: I got shelled, and I couldn't get in my car fast enough to come home and begin plotting a new life.

But George Bamberger, our pitching coach, was trying to convince me to go to the Puerto Rican Winter League and work out my problems. I fought him all the way. "If I can't get the hitters out in the Instructional League, what will happen to me in Puerto Rico when I face major-leaguers?" I said.

George wouldn't take no. "You haven't pitched in two years," he told me, "and if you want to come back to the big leagues, you have to keep working at it. Besides, what have you got to lose?"

At the same time a friend in Baltimore suggested that I try an anti-inflammatory drug to help cure my arm problem. I finally heeded Bamberger's advice and went to Puerto Rico. The drug helped to cure my arm and, free to pitch without pain, I got my rhythm back. The following season I led the American League in won-lost percentage (.800) with a 16–4 record, including my no-hitter.

If George hadn't stayed with me, I don't believe I could have achieved such a sudden turnabout and restarted my career with such continued good results.

Perhaps that is the closest I ever came to failing or quitting, yet every time I lost a game, in effect I failed—and, as I noted, I had 152 of them. Losing was one of the toughest things for a pitcher, at least for me, to get over. If I lost on Sunday, then I had four days to live with it, and if I lost in my next start on Thursday, then I really started to worry about it. The worst ones were the close games because, no matter how well I prepared, I still replayed that game, looking to find the thing that had beaten me. Conversely, if I was beaten badly, I went right home and went to sleep.

But the key really is not to dwell on the failures, because that only heightens the stress that naturally comes with wanting to succeed. Again, if you prepared well and failed, you must find con-solation in having given it your best shot. Do the

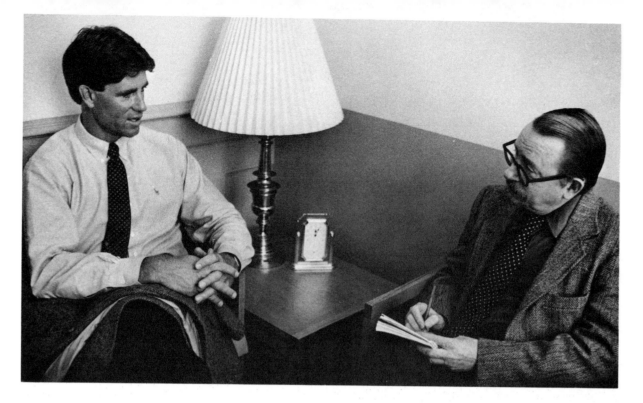

same thing the next time and you are apt to succeed.

To understand a problem, I always believed you must know its causes, and wanting to succeed isn't a bad place to begin. All of us want success in some measure and for reasons such as fame, money, personal satisfaction or all of them. There are people who are totally intoxicated with succeeding and will do anything—fair or foul—to achieve it. There also are people who will work with all of their talents to achieve it; and there are others who really want it but either don't know how to go about achieving it or really aren't motivated to pay whatever price is necessary.

All of us probably fall into one of those broad categories, and without trying any instant psycho-analysis, I know that I forced myself to succeed in a high-tension business. Yet I had only one headache during my entire career, and I awoke with that on the day I started my first All-Star game. It turned out to be my best All-Star performance.

Tension, or stress, strikes each of us in different ways. When Steve Stone pitched for us, he said the most tension-free day he enjoyed was the day he pitched. I always felt the opposite, but much of that, I believe, had to do with the expectation level. Except for the 1980 season, when he won the Cy Young Award, Steve basically was a .500 pitcher, so no one had great

expectations of him when he pitched. Jim Palmer was expected to win twenty games—by others and by himself. I always felt that if I won nineteen games, then I'd had a bad season. Pure and simple, that is self-induced pressure, and much of the pressure we face in our daily lives comes from within. Sure, you can have a demanding boss who never lets up in what he expects from you, but remember, you can only work to your capabilities. If you work, or compete, to the utmost of your ability, then no one can expect anything more. If those expectations become too unreasonable, then you must reevaluate what you are doing and how you can do it more comfortably and not live in a world of unreasonable stress.

That does not mean that you have failed—no one fails who does his best. It simply means that you either must speak up and let it be known that you can do no more than your best, or else look for another situation where those efforts will be appreciated and rewarded. That is one big reason why players in professional sports seek to be traded; and, conversely, many are traded because they don't work to their potential.

Some days when I pitched I was almost untouchable. There also were days when I simply did not feel right from the moment I got out of bed that morning, and then I struggled. Sometimes I got through all right; sometimes I didn't. Yet I wouldn't accept in my own mind that I couldn't always be invincible, and obviously I added more stress to my own life.

I tried to compensate, at least in my own mind, by working harder and harder to condition myself. Finally, our team orthopedist a few years back said to me, "Jim, you can't do any more exercises, either preventive or corrective, because you've done them all."

Certainly I was the cause of my own anxieties, and it wasn't until about ten years into my career that I realized that baseball is a team game, and that as a pitcher I had to go out and perform my job like anyone else. I couldn't win games by myself, though as a pitcher I was the key ingredient. As I said, there were nights when I was about 95 percent of the game, and if I got one or two runs, it was all over.

But in the biggest percentage of the games I was just out there doing my job, trying to hold the opposition to two or three runs, or close enough so that our guys could get enough runs to win.

The key: You can't do it all by yourself, but you can do enough by being yourself, and, in the end, that is winning.

Win ... succeed ... call it what you wish, but that is the ultimate end of everything we do. It only happens if you give it your best shot, and even then there are no guarantees. I know it sounds trite, but you can't ever give up; you have to keep searching for a way to be successful that works within your capabilities and within your personality.

That brings up another key point: Don't try to be someone or something that isn't really you. Sooner or later the real you will shine through and you will then be tabbed as a phony, and any respect you have generated will disappear. Athletes, particularly those playing team sports, are adept at spotting phonies because we have played for so many different types of people during our careers. Earl Weaver, Ralph Houk, Sparky Anderson and Walter Alston all were great managers, but if someone went out and tried to copy their style without having their talent or personality, that person would fail. You can only be yourself. And you will make life a lot easier to live by not always having to rememer who you are trying to copy.

And be honest in all of your dealings. I've always said that honesty may have been my biggest failing because I never hid my feelings about what I considered something of importance to our team and to my own career. That is one form of honesty; and the other is to be honest with yourself by doing your best.

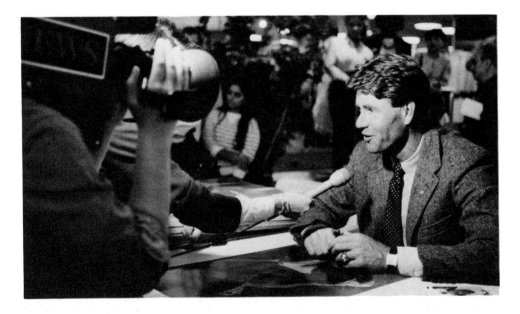

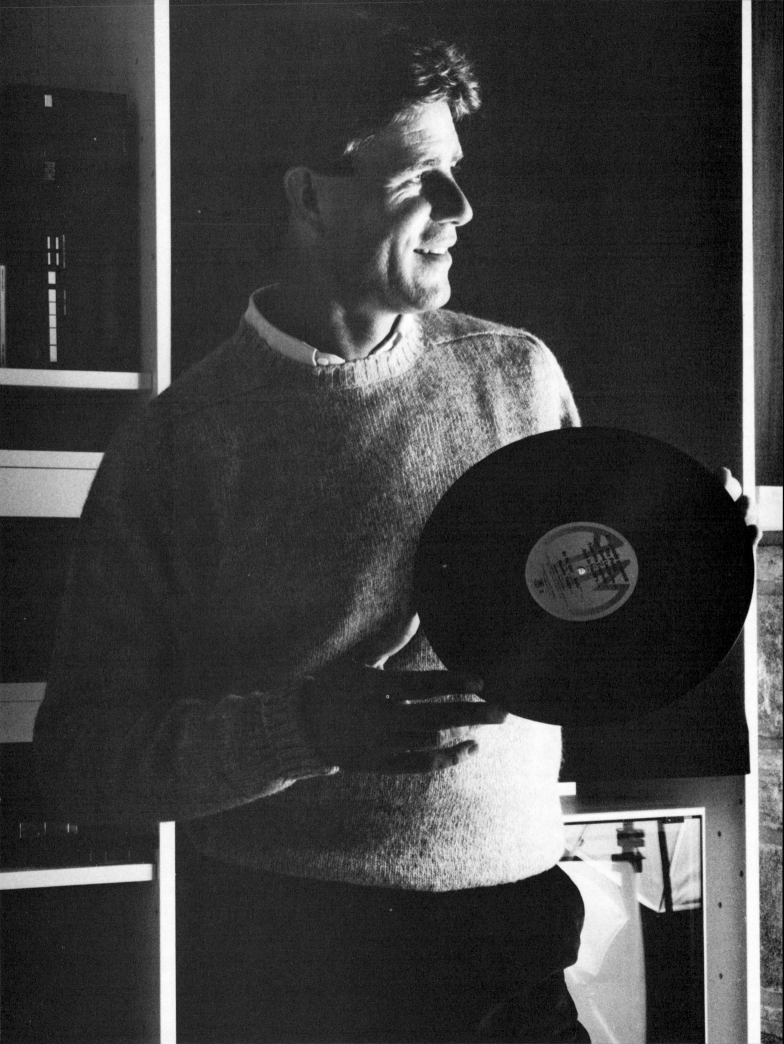

EPILOGUE:
JIM PALMER—THE PRIVATE PERSON,
THE PUBLIC PERFORMER

Just who is this man Jim Palmer who has given you his formula for a more fulfilling lifestyle?

Certainly you have known that he was without peer during most of his nineteen major-league seasons with the Baltimore Orioles, and perhaps after reading this book and learning more about the manner in which he directs his life, you can understand how much of this success came about.

Jim was born with tremendous physical abilities, but, unlike many others who are similarly blessed, he worked to perfect and use those abilities to the very utmost. It is obvious from his thoughts that he is a very disciplined and single-minded person who allows no one, or nothing, to block his path to self-fulfillment. This is the singular quality which all of life's great achievers—athlete and non-athlete alike—have in common.

I have known and worked with other athletes and coaches whose achievements in their par-ticular sports are as great as Palmer's, and in every one I see a bit of Jim Palmer; and in Jim Palmer I see a lot of them.

But as much as Jim and his ilk are super-achievers, they are first and foremost people like you and me, and they must live life away from the arena, coping, as we all must, with what is dished up to them. There is no better way to get a glimpse of how someone handles this part of living than to see him at home, where the glitter and glitz of public life are shed for the plain garb that tags him simply as a person.

My previous experience with Jim before I began helping him to compile the material for this book consisted wholly of interviews after games when the Orioles played in Boston and I was working as a writer-columnist for the *Boston Herald Traveler*. That had been more than a decade ago, and since then I had seen and heard him in other interview sessions, and I had read about his career as it spiraled to such great heights. The solidly positive

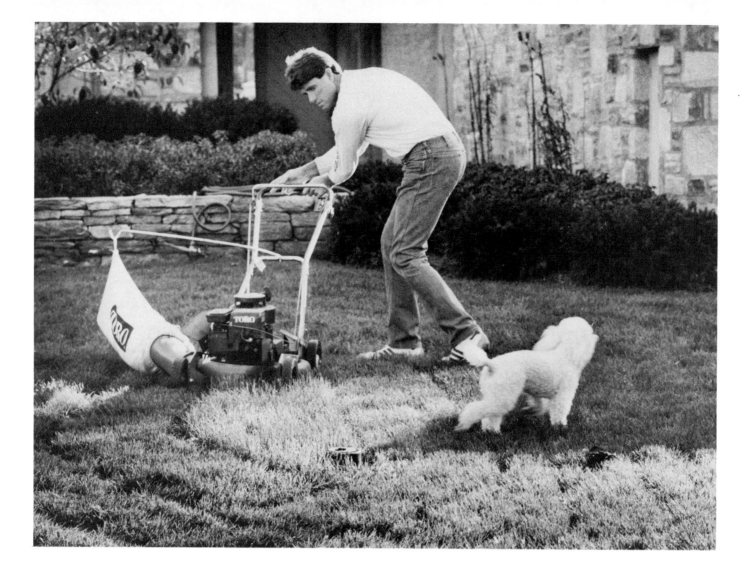

impressions from those early interview sessions were never lessened.

But journalists rarely are afforded a look at their subject away from his venue, so my perceptions were open to all that might pass before me during our sessions together. And what I found was most pleasing and fulfilled a shadowy impression I had that Jim Palmer really was about how he seemed in public...a good person whom you would want as a friend...who was strong in his beliefs yet easygoing in his manner...and who was eminently perceptive about the world as it pertained to him, past, present and future.

His home, set in a newly built area in one of Baltimore's northern suburbs, is nestled next to similar homes whose occupants pursue a variety of occupations. Hence, Jim has become part of a community that accepts him for what he is, and while aware of who he is, it has made him one of their own.

Inside his home there is a wide-open feeling of comfort and an informality that is a direct reflection of his real personality, yet with no visible evidence that he was one of baseball's greatest pitchers. Jim always has nurtured deep affection for the West, where he spent most of his youth, and the paintings and wall hangings are visible mementoes of those memories.

From sunup to sunset, Jim never stops.

He and his home are strangers to each other for a good part of the year while he travels in his role as Jockey's spokesman, as a sportscaster for ABC and in sundry other ventures which trade off his personal popularity for some commercial interest. But when he is home, there is almost a

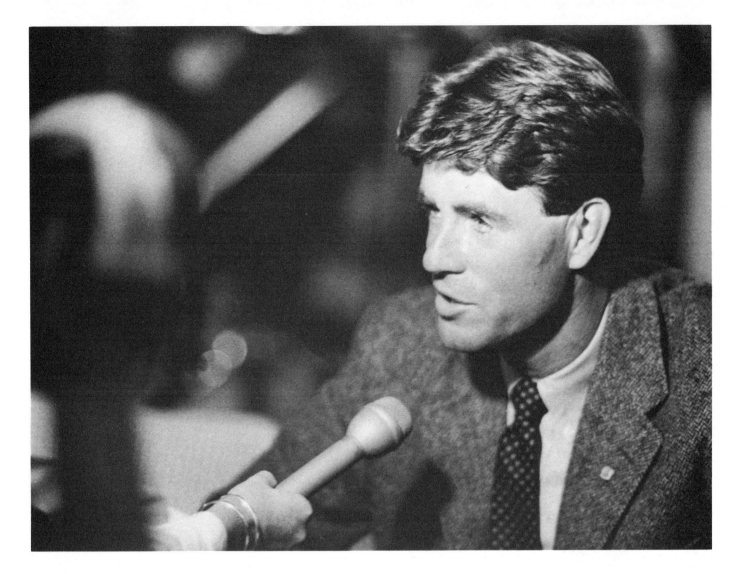

dervishness that sends him whisking to and fro around that home, with his sophisticated stereo system blaring out everything from "The William Tell Overture" to Gershwin's "Rhapsody in Blue" to The Police.

From sunup to sunset, Jim never stops. In the good weather he will be outside cutting his own lawn and then caring for that of a neighbor as a gesture of gratitude for the man's looking after his home while he is gone. He attacks the intruders which grow in his garden with the same intensity with which he backed down some of baseball's best hitters, and takes pride in having his property always looking its best.

Last summer, for example, after having been away for nearly three weeks on assignment at the Olympic Games for ABC, a friend asked how he planned to relax after such a long absence. He expected that Jim might talk about just kicking off his shoes and putting his feet on a stool beneath

one of the shade trees in his yard. The jolt came when Palmer very matter-of-factly pointed out that he had neglected his yard and garden and had "at least a day's work facing me to try and catch up." So much for goofing off.

Living alone, except for the times when his two teenage daughters, Jamie and Kelly, come to spend time, he is the total domestic. He washes and folds his own laundry, and if necessary, he will haul out the iron and ironing board and use them with a skill many men might envy. He does his own food-shopping, often late in the evening when his favorite supermarket is uncrowded, and if a neighbor or friend needs something, too, consider it done.

Palmer also does his own cooking, and is not afraid to try something in one of the half-dozen cookbooks which adorn a shelf above his sink. We have seen how careful he is in his choice of food, but that doesn't mean he won't tackle a *coq au vin*

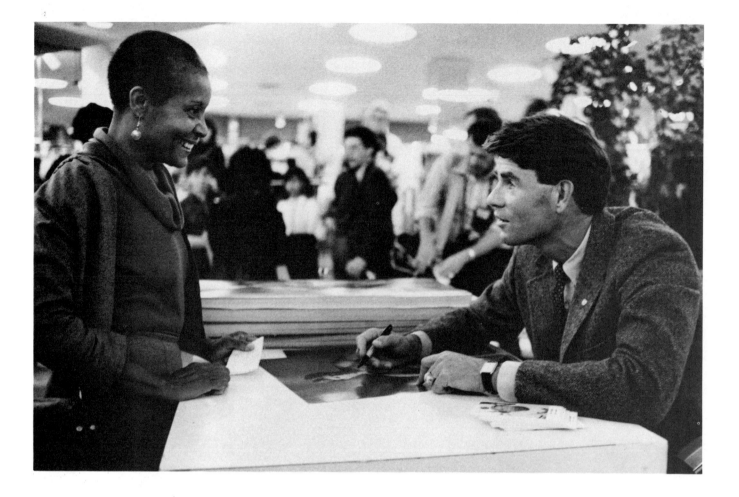

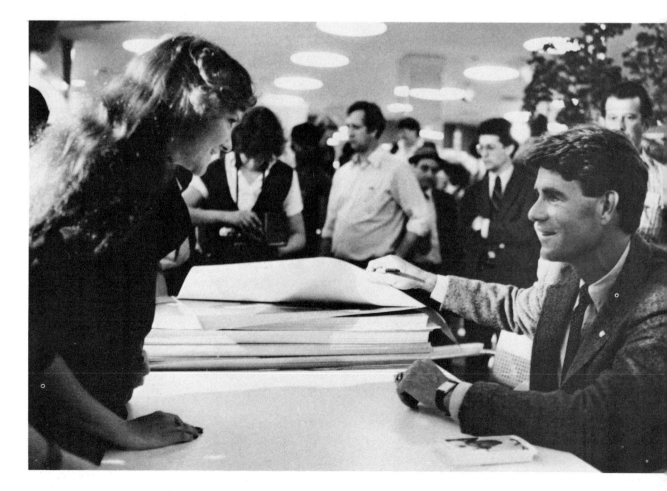

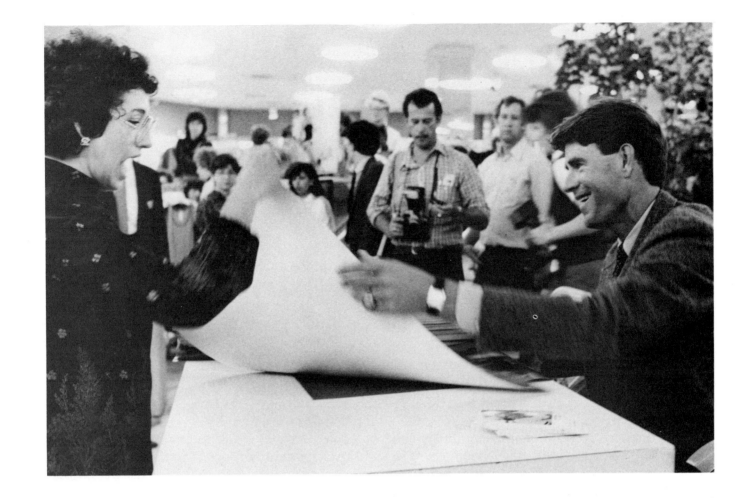

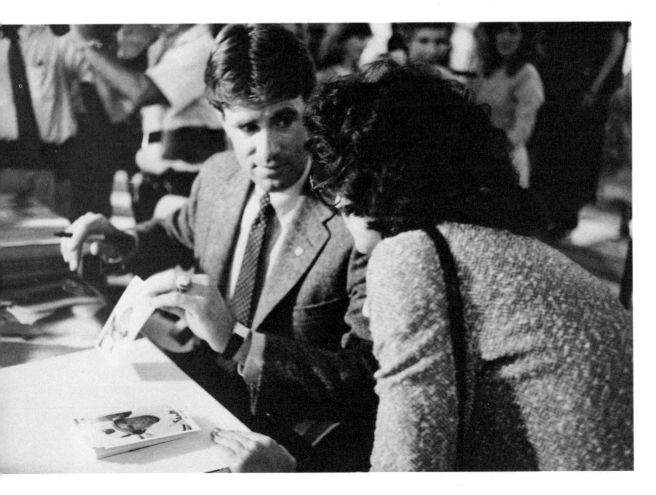

for the first time, or be a willing participant in a gala pre-opera dinner party.

Those who know him well say that he is one of the world's great "neatniks," that everything has its place and is kept there. Order is the key, but that should not surprise anyone because it was the way he maintained his baseball life.

His telephone is forever busy, and when he is not attending to his home, or to his personal business, he will be meeting friends for racquetball, or tennis, or for a game of golf...provided, of course, that he is not riding his ten-speed racing bike or doing a bit of jogging.

When he walks, he ambles along in big strides, head often tilted to one side as he considers his route.

This energy consumption is not totally frenetic, and while Jim must be forever busy, it is done with an ease and direction that mark the easy-going side of his personality. When he walks, he ambles along in big strides, head often tilted to one side as he considers his route. Yet his lankiness seems to cover great gobs of territory in a minimum of time because his internal compass has been set, the route charted and there is little need to dally.

It is marvelous to watch him when his two daughters, both blonde and with an emerging beauty that will soon have a head-turning quality, come into his life. Here, Jim is dear old Dad, who is sometimes peppered with exclamations of amazement at being so...well, fatherish as he suggests that yes, homework is more important than talking on the phone; or that a slight weight problem isn't solved by complaining about it, but by doing something about it.

The chatter is incessant and he revels in the little teasing challenges which are tossed his way and which he tosses back. Yet he also will stand on a cold, wind-swept plain to watch his girls play after-school sports and he will patiently accompany his oldest as she begins seeking a college to continue her education.

He never says so, but he fairly bursts with good feeling when, seeing him alone as she heads out for an evening of fun, one of the girls nudges up and says, "Oh, Daddy, you're alone. I'll stay with you."

"Don't be silly," he says. "I'll be fine. Go have a good time."

He also chuckles when his other daughter, seeing him alone, gives a big wave—"See you, Dad"—and is off on her own mission.

At night, while the beautiful people of the world who are often linked with him in display advertising are amusing themselves, Jim may sit at his butcher-block kitchen table and read the newspaper or peruse one of the many magazines, such as *Architectural Digest,* to which he subscribes. He may retire to his office/den in the rear of his home, where only two of his four Gold Glove awards are displayed as the only evidence of his baseball greatness, and catch up on some work.

Not truly exciting in the real sense of the word, but that is Jim Palmer. When he works with a collaborator, he is clear in his thoughts, articulate and perceptive in disseminating his ideas. He shows a vital interest in all that is about him, whether or not that is the subject of the moment. He certainly knows who he was as a major-league player, and his career is carefully crystallized within his memory so he can cite season records, games and individual incidents which help to illustrate his points.

Yet he is not so caught up with himself that he can ever ignore those who play different roles in his life. During outdoor photo sessions for this book, he once cautioned those who worked with him to be most considerate of his neighbors lest they regard him as too overbearing; and in a session at a private school near his home, he openly fretted that the crew was impeding access to the main property, and that cars parked off the road should be carefully driven away lest the soft grass be churned up, leaving scars.

In reality, the young people and their parents were so surprised to see Jim working in the photography session that they deliberately slowed, waved and in some instances shouted their affection. He just waved back and with the natural shy manner, so accentuated by his boyish good

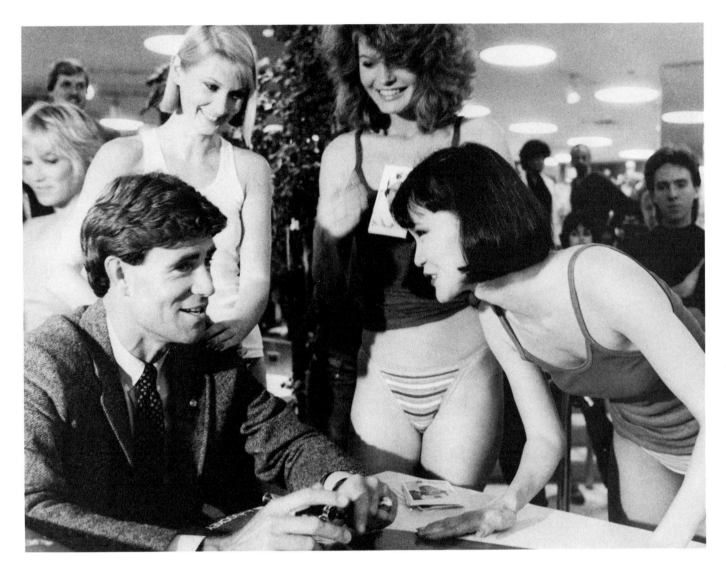

looks, probably reinforced their affection for him.

That affection, of course, has grown around Baltimore because of his tremendous contributions to the community, both as an athlete and in his untiring work with the Cystic Fibrosis Research Foundation for over thirteen years, mostly as its national sports chairman.

The adulation of Oriole fans is well founded on his achievements on the playing field—268 victories from 1965 thru 1984, including a no-hitter back in 1969 against the Oakland A's only four days after coming off a six-week period on the disabled list; five one-hitters; eleven two-hitters; and eighteen three-hitters. He finished his career with a club record of 2,212 strikeouts over 3,949 innings pitched, and during all of that he

recorded fifty-three shutouts. He also won the American League's Cy Young Award three times, in 1973, 1975, and 1976, as well as the aforementioned four Gold Glove awards as the league's best fielding pitcher, 1976–79.

In post-season play he became the youngest pitcher ever to hurl a shutout in the World Series when he beat the Los Angeles Dodgers and their great left-hander, Sandy Koufax, in 1966. Jim was just ten days shy of his twenty-first birthday. His sixteen wins that year, his second full season in the major leagues, helped the Orioles to their first pennant and, subsequently, their first world championship.

Jim pitched in five other World Series for an overall 4–2 record. In addition, he won four or

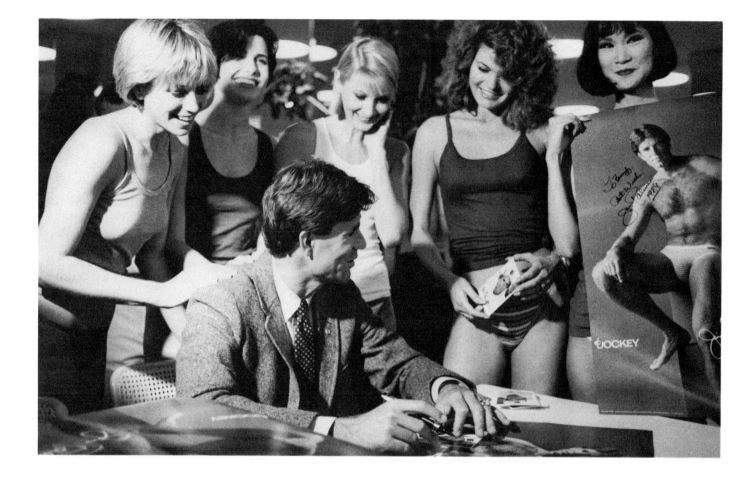

five decisions in the American League's Championship Series over six different seasons with a splendid 1.96 earned-run average and pitched in five All-Star games in the six times he was selected for that honor.

During the seventies, there was no better right-handed pitcher in the American League.

During the seventies there was no better right-handed pitcher in the American League, and some of the marks he has left behind bear testimony to that achievement:

- He led the American League in won-lost percentage twice—1969 (.800 on 16–4 record) and 1982 (.750 on 15–5).

- He pitched a club-record ten shutouts for the Orioles in 1975.
- In a five-game stretch in 1978 he had four shutouts, including three in a row.
- He pitched back-to-back shutouts six times in his career.
- He never gave up a grand-slam home run during regular-season and championship play.

Away from baseball, Jim was one of Arizona's greatest schoolboy athletes while at Scottsdale High School, winning all-state honors in baseball, football and basketball, and then had his choice of receiving a college scholarship for any of the three sports. He began working as a sports rep for Jockey underwear products in 1980, and in 1983 he received the American Image Award given by the Male Apparel Industry and Men's Fashion Association of America.

His major-league baseball career now is behind him and obviously the last plateau will come in a few years on a warm summer afternoon in Cooperstown, New York, when he is inducted into Baseball's Hall of Fame, which is all but a foregone conclusion once the five-year waiting period has ended.

Ahead lie various career choices and all of the indecisions and crises which accompany life in the world of commerce and industry. Already proficient as a color commentator for ABC's playoff and World Series telecasts, and having delved into other broadcast opportunities, Jim has said that he wants more for his life than just a one-dimensional occupation.

There is little doubt that if he cares to harness the same mental energy that drove him to such great heights as an athlete, and couples it with the drive and single-minded determination that were his baseball hallmarks, then Jim Palmer will continue his success on other levels. He has only to follow the precepts which he has laid down in this book to keep him on that path.

I'm betting he will.

Jack Clary
Stow, Massachusetts
November 1984

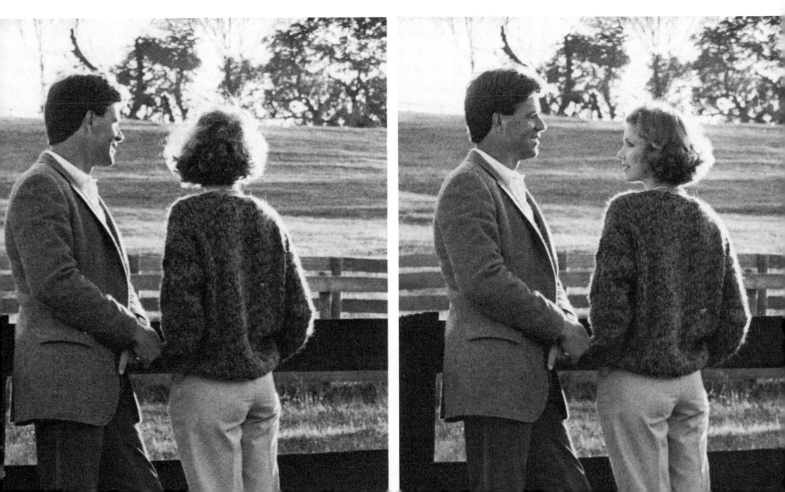

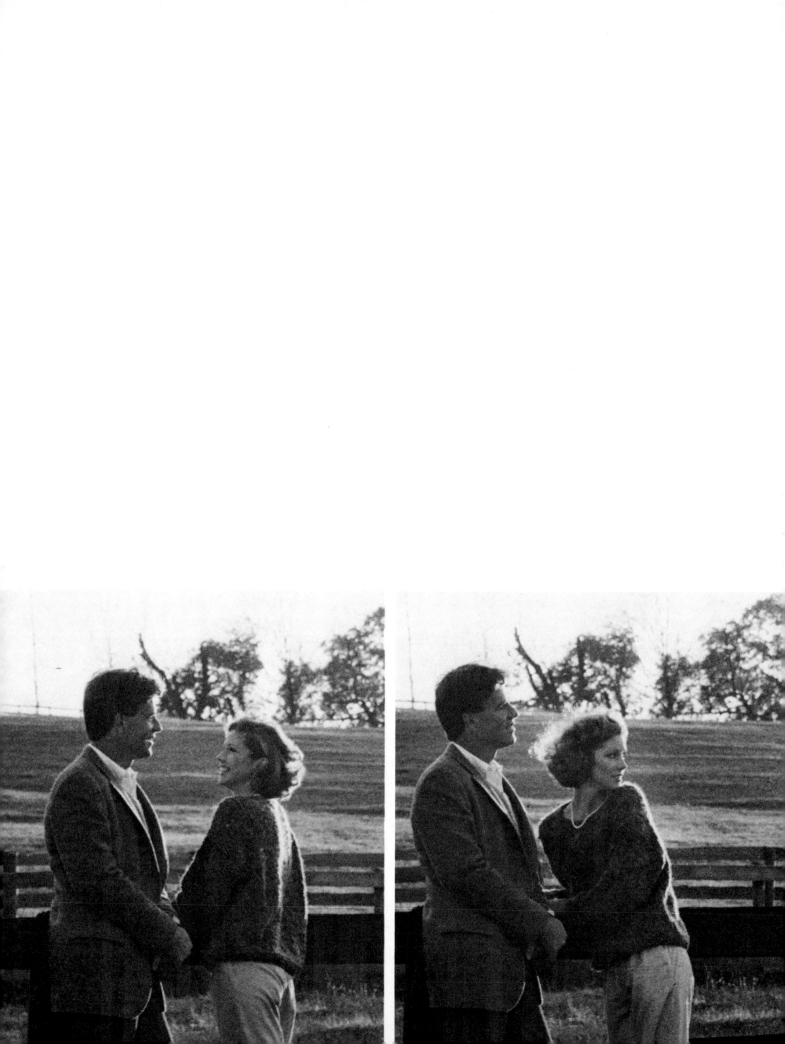

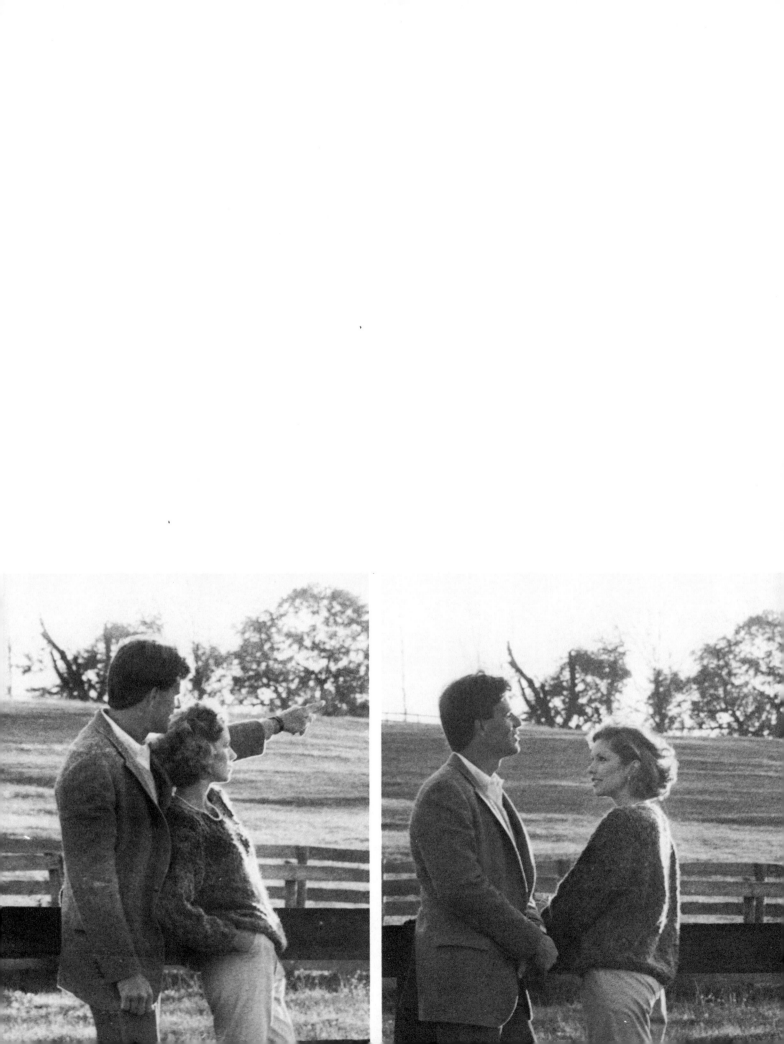

JIM PALMER'S MAJOR LEAGUE RECORD

YEAR CLUB	W-L	ERA	G	GS	CG	SHO	SV	IP	H	BB	SO
1964 Aberdeen—1	11- 3	2.51	19	19	9	4	..	129	75	130	107
1965 Baltimore	5- 4	3.72	27	6	0	0	..	92	75	56	75
1966 Baltimore	15-10	3.46	30	30	6	0	..	208	176	91	147
1967 Baltimore	3- 1	2.94	9	9	2	1	..	49	34	20	23
Rochester	0- 0	11.57	2	2	0	0	..	7	12	5	6
Miami	1- 1	2.00	5	5	0	0	..	27	20	10	16
1968 Elmira	0- 2	4.32	6	6	0	0	..	25	18	19	26
Rochester	0- 0	13.50	2	2	0	0	..	4	4	8	6
Miami	0- 0	0.00	2	2	0	0	..	8	4	9	5
1969 Baltimore	16- 4	2.34	26	23	11	6	0	181	131	64	123
1970 Baltimore	20-10	2.71	39	39	17	•5	0	•305	263	100	199
1971 Baltimore	20- 9	2.68	37	37	20	3	0	282	231	106	184
1972 Baltimore	21-10	2.07	36	36	18	3	0	274	219	70	184
1973 Baltimore	22- 9	*2.40	38	37	19	6	1	296	225	113	158
1974 Baltimore	7-12	3.27	26	26	5	2	0	179	176	69	84
1975 Baltimore	•23-11	*2.09	39	38	25	*10	1	323	253	80	193
1976 Baltimore	*22-13	2.51	*40	40	23	6	0	*315	255	84	159
1977 Baltimore	•20-11	2.91	39	*39	•22	3	0	*319	263	99	193
1978 Baltimore	21-12	2.46	38	38	19	6	0	*296	246	97	138
1979 Baltimore	10- 6	3.29	23	22	7	0	0	156	144	43	67
1980 Baltimore	16-10	3.98	34	33	4	0	0	224	238	74	109
1981 Baltimore	7- 8	3.75	22	22	5	0	0	127	117	46	35
1982 Baltimore	15- 5	3.13	36	32	8	2	1	227	195	63	103
1983 Baltimore	5- 4	4.23	14	11	0	0	0	76.2	86	19	34
Hagerstown—2	2- 0	3.46	2	2	0	0	0	13	13	2	11
1984 Baltimore	0- 3	9.17	5		0	0	0	17.2	22	17	4
M.L. Totals	268-152	2.87	558		518	211	53	3947.2	3349	1311	2212

*Led league   •Tied for league lead
 1—Signed by Baltimore organization as free agent on 8/16/63
 2—On rehabilitation assignment, Aug. 6-12, 1983.

Common Muscle Discomforts

Many people think that if you don't feel stiff and sore after a day of exercising, you haven't worked hard enough. These people do not understand that proper exercising is started slowly and intensified only over a long period of time. Unfortunately, overwork and too much enthusiasm in the beginning result in muscle soreness and poor performance on the following days.

Muscle soreness is but one of the injuries commonly encountered by participants in exercising and sports activities. The descriptions that follow are a guide for identifying the nature of the discomfort and relieving it through proven first-aid treatment. Lesser injuries can be safely treated by following these simple directions. More serious injuries, or those that result in extreme loss of motion of the muscles and joints, should be examined by a doctor.

General Muscle Soreness

This is a feeling of stiffness and aching in the muscles, usually experienced twelve to twenty-four hours after a workout. The condition occurs in almost everyone who works out, even in trained athletes. It always follows the first workout of an inactive person.

When exercise is resumed the day after soreness sets in, it will cause pain; this usually disappears after two to three minutes of activity. When the exercising is ended, however, the soreness reappears to a lesser degree.

Soreness can be minimized by a progressive series of exercises, calling for harder workouts after periods of milder ones, and by adequate tapering-off of the exercise program each day.

One of the by-products of muscle-exercising is

lactic acid. If it is not removed from the cells by tapering-off methods, muscle soreness results. If a regular program of exercise is maintained for at least two weeks, this type of soreness will gradually disappear. It usually takes this long for the skeletal-muscular system to become accustomed to the workout.

Muscle Cramps

These are prolonged, painful contractions of one or more muscles. They are most often experienced in the legs or feet. Flexing and massage will help to alleviate the condition and restore the muscle to the near-normal state of tension.

Inadequate warmup is one cause of cramps; also, there is some evidence that improper diet contributes to their occurrence. If the condition of cramps occurs on a regular basis, a physician should be consulted.

Sprains

A sprain involves the twisting of a joint, with subsequent tearing and stretching of the ligaments supporting the joint. A severe sprain often involves injury to the surrounding nerves and muscles.

The treatment is ice application, followed by an x-ray to determine the extent of the injury. Heat is not applied to a sprain for at least thirty-six hours after the injury. A sprain should always be referred to a doctor for complete diagnosis and treatment.

Strains

A strain involves the actual tearing of a muscle fiber. The seriousness of the injury depends on the amount of fibers involved in the tear.

This overstretching of the muscle fibers is often the result of a maximum effort without proper warmup. To remember how your muscles react when properly warmed up, consider the modest analogy between muscle fibers and taffy. After having been kneaded and stretched, a piece of taffy is capable of maximum tensions and twisting without tearing. Try the twisting and pulling when it is cold, and it will break. Your muscles respond the same way; extend them when they are cold, and they will tear and rupture.

Athletes commonly refer to strains as "pulled muscles" or "muscle pulls." When use of the strained, or "pulled," muscle is required, there is severe discomfort and pain. The treatment is the immediate application of ice to reduce the swelling and capillary bleeding. After thirty-six hours heat may be applied. When possible the injury should be protected against further injury by adhesive taping. Immediate resumption of activity is not recommended, as the weaker fibrous scar-tissue, which is replacing the torn muscle, is prone to further injury.

Contusions

A contusion is the result of a blow to some portion of the body, causing tissue-tearing and hemorrhaging. The injured area appears red and swollen; the muscle is usually immobilized after a short time. Contusions are common to the quadriceps (or thighs) and are referred to as "charley horses."

Handball players who play without proper gloves often experience contusions of the palm. This is caused by the constant striking of the soft tissues of the hand by the hard rubber ball. By soaking the hand in cold water, temporary relief from the soreness may be achieved.

The immediate treatment of any contusion should be to pack it with ice. After thirty-six hours heat should be applied; this will help to speed up the absorption of the swelling. An examination by a doctor is recommended in order to determine the extent of deep tissue damage.

Calorie Chart

Type of Food	Amount	Calories
Breads and Cereals		
Biscuit	1 medium	130
Bread		
white	1 slice	60
whole wheat	1 slice	55
Corn flakes	1 cup	85
Muffin, corn	1	135
Pancake	1 thin, medium	60
Roll, sweet	1 medium	200
Waffle	1 medium	215
Beverages		
Alcoholic		
beer	12-ounce bottle	170
gin	1 jigger	105
martini	1 cocktail glass	145
whiskey	1 jigger	105
wine, port	1 wine glass	160

Type of Food	Amount	Calories
Carbonated cola-type drink	6 ounces	60
Cocoa, with whole milk	1 cup	236
Coffee, black	1 cup	0
Ice-cream soda, vanilla	1½ cups	260
Malted milk-shake, chocolate	1½ cups	500
Milk		
skim or buttermilk	1 cup	86
whole	1 cup	166
Tea		
plain	1 cup	0
with light cream (1 tablespoon)	1 cup	35
with sugar (1 teaspoon)	1 cup	15

Candy

Candy bar, milk chocolate	1 bar (2 ounces)	290
Chocolate creams	2 average	110
Fudge	1 piece (1-inch square)	115
Jelly beans	5	35

Desserts

Brownies	1 piece, 2 × 2 × ¾ inches	140
Cake		
angel food	2-inch wedge	110
chocolate, 2 layers	2-inch wedge	420
plain, 2 layers, iced	2-inch wedge	320
pound	1 slice	130
Cookies, assorted	1 cookie, 3″ diameter	110
Cupcake, iced	1	160
Custard, baked	½ cup	140
Doughnut, raised	1 average	120
Fig bar	1 small	55
Gelatin dessert, plain	½ cup	80
Ice, fruit	½ cup	75
Ice cream		
chocolate	½ cup	175
vanilla	½ cup	150
Pie		
apple	4-inch wedge	330
lemon meringue	4-inch wedge	300
pumpkin	4-inch wedge	265
Pudding, vanilla	½ cup	140
Sherbet	½ cup	120
Sundae, chocolate	½ cup ice cream and 2 tablespoons sauce	330

Type of Food	Amount	Calories
Dressings		
Blue cheese	1 tablespoon	90
French	1 tablespoon	60
Mayonnaise	1 tablespoon	110
Salad oil	1 tablespoon	125
Thousand island	1 tablespoon	75
Fish and Seafood		
Clams	6	90
Crab meat	½ cup	90
Lobster	½ cup	90
Mackerel	1 piece, 4 × 3 × ½ inches	200
Salmon, broiled	1 piece	205
Sardines	5-7 medium	180
Shrimp, cooked	12	165
Tuna, canned in oil	½ cup	215
Fruits and Juices		
Apple	1 medium	75
Apricots, fresh	1 medium	18
Avocado	½ peeled	185
Banana	1 medium	90
Blueberries, fresh	1 cup	45
Cantaloupe	½ medium	37
Cherries, fresh	½ cup	30
Cranberry sauce	1 tablespoon	30
Dates, fresh	¼ cup	125
Figs, dried	1	60
Grapefruit	½ medium	75
Grapefruit juice	½ cup	65
Grapes	40	105
Honeydew melon	1 wedge	50
Orange	1 medium	70
Orange juice	½ cup fresh	58
Peach, fresh	1 medium	35
Pear	1 medium	95
Pineapple, crushed	½ cup	100
Pineapple juice	½ cup	65
Plums, fresh	1 medium	30
Prunes	½ cup	150
Raisins	¼ cup	215
Raspberries, red, fresh	½ cup	35
Strawberries, fresh	1 cup	60
Tangerines	1 medium	40
Watermelon	1 wedge, 4 × 8 inches	120

Type of Food	Amount	Calories
Meat		
Bacon	4 strips	380
Beef		
chuck	6 ounces	530
rib roast	2 thin slices, 4 × 3 inches	280
Chicken		
dark meat, fried	drumstick and thigh	245
pot pie	8 ounces	485
white meat, fried	½ breast	215
Frankfurter	2	310
Ham, cooked	2 slices 7 × 2 inches	250
Lamb chops	2	280
Liver, beef, fried	1 thin slice	120
Meat loaf	2 slices	230
Pork chop	2	260
Sausage, pork	1 link	95
Spareribs	4 ribs	330
Steak		
round	6 ounces	400
sirloin	6 ounces	510
Turkey	average serving	246
Veal	1 piece	185
Other Dishes		
Beef stew and vegetables	1 cup	252
Chili with beans	½ cup	170
Eggs		
boiled	1	80
omelet	2 eggs	270
poached	1	80
scrambled	1	110
Macaroni and cheese	½ cup	240
Pizza, cheese	4-inch wedge	185
Sandwiches		
bacon, lettuce and tomato	average	280
ham	average	280
hamburger	average	330
hot dog with bun	average	280
peanut butter	average	330
Spaghetti, Italian	1 cup	331
Snacks and Appetizers		
Almonds	5	40
Cashews	1 ounce (8 nuts)	164

Type of Food	Amount	Calories
Peanut brittle	1 piece	85
Peanuts, shelled	15-17	85
Pecans	1 tablespoon, chopped	52
Popcorn, buttered	1 cup	90
Potato chips	10 chips	110
Pretzels	5 small sticks	20

Soups

Beef	1 cup	100
Clam chowder	1 cup	85
Cream soups (celery, mushroom)	1 cup	200
Potato	1 cup	185
Tomato	1 cup	90
Vegetable	1 cup	80

Spreads

Jam	1 tablespoon	55
Jelly	1 tablespoon	50
Maple syrup	1 tablespoon	50
Peanut butter	1 tablespoon	90
Preserves	1 tablespoon	55

Vegetables

Asparagus	½ cup	20
Beans, cooked		
green	½ cup	15
lima	½ cup	75
snap	½ cup	15
wax	½ cup	15
yellow	½ cup	15
Beets	½ cup	35
Broccoli	½ cup	20
Cabbage	½ cup	20
Carrots		
cooked	½ cup	20
raw	5-inch piece	20
Cauliflower, cooked	½ cup	15
Celery, raw	4 5-inch stalks	12
Corn		
on cob	1 medium ear	65
cooked	½ cup	80
Cucumber	6 slices	5
Lettuce	2 large leaves	5
Onions, cooked	½ cup	40

Type of Food	Amount	Calories
Peas, cooked	½ cup	60
Potato		
baked	1 medium	96
French-fried	10 medium	155
mashed	1 cup	120
Radishes, raw	4 small	10
Sauerkraut	½ cup	15
Spinach, cooked	½ cup	20
Sweet potatoes		
baked	1 average	250
candied	1 medium	300
Tomatoes, fresh	1 medium	30

Miscellaneous

Butter	1 tablespoon	100
Margarine	1 tablespoon	100
Olive, green	1 large	10
Pickle, dill	1 large	15
Sugar	1 tablespoon	48
Whipped cream	1 tablespoon	48

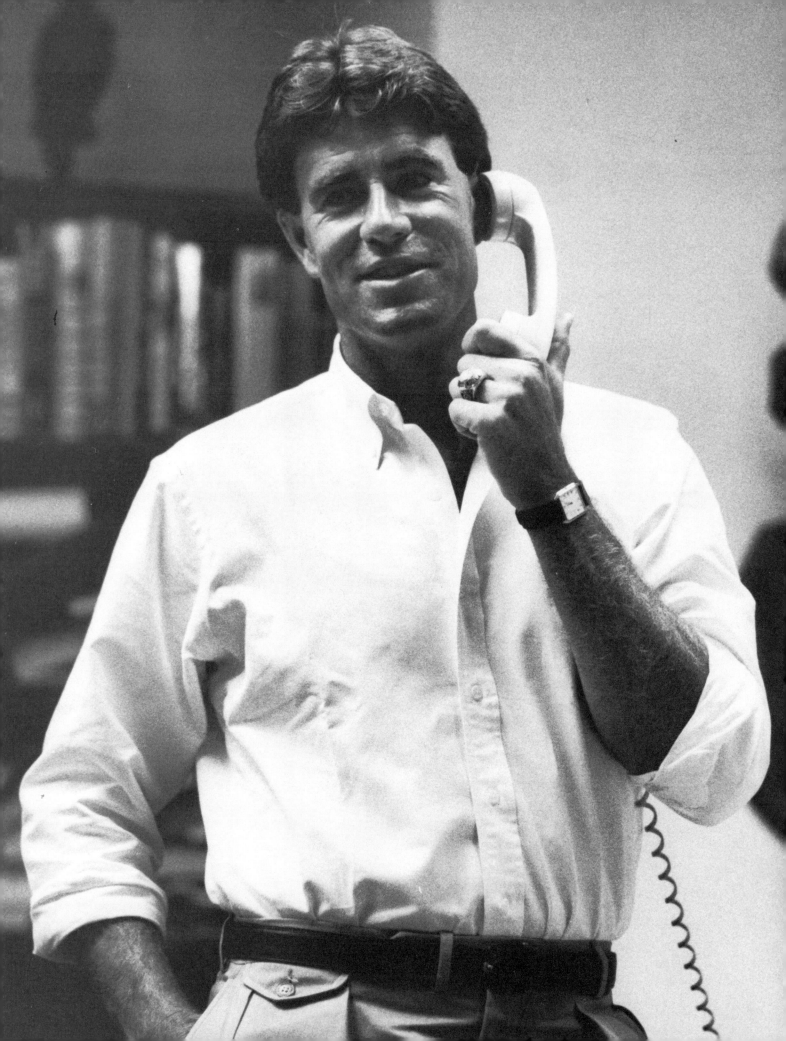

INDEX

Abdominal muscles, 71
  sit-ups and, 20
Achilles' tendon stretch, 16
Aerobic exercises, 30
  definition of, 8
Aging, 80
Airplane stretch, 13, 15
Alcohol, 88–89
Anaerobic exercises, 8
Anderson, Sparky, 126
Ankle circle, 38, 40
Arm circle, 26, 27
  reverse, 26, 27
Arm crossover, 45, 46
Arm swing, circular, 42
Ascorbic acid, 85
Atherosclerosis, cholesterol and, 82

Back
  alignment of, 70
  body mechanics and, 73–74
  flat, 71
  postural problems and, 72–73
Back arm reach, 72
  palms turned in, 38, 41
  palms turned out, 38, 41

Back extensor muscles, 71
Back leg lift
  bent knee, 23, 25
  straight knee, 23, 25
Back lift, 26
Backpacking, 57
Back stretch, 18, 19, 73
Balance, body, 69–75
Baldness, 103–4
Ball roll, 48
Bamberger, George, 127
Barbell arms, 22, 24
Baseball, 1–2, 57, 88, 139–41
  stress in, 121–29
Basketball, 56–57
Bauer, Hank, 109
B-complex vitamins, 84
Bends
  neck, 12
  side, 13, 14, 73
Bent knee-up, 20, 21
Biceps raise, 29, 30
Bicycling, 54, 56–58
Body balance, 69–75
Body lotion, 95, 98
Body mechanics, 73–74

Body types, 111–12
Bow and arrow, 22
Bowling, 56, 58
Breathing, stretching and, 12

Caffeine, 88, 89
Calories, 81
Canoe, 58
Carbohydrates, 83
Carrying, 74
Chin tuck, 72
Cholesterol, 82
Circular arm swing, 42
Climbing, 57
Clothes, 107–15
    body types and, 11–12
    care of, 116
    for cycling, 54
    dress code of Baltimore Orioles, 107, 109, 111
    for running, 52
    for semiformal (business) occasions, 114–16
    for sports and leisure wear, 116
    for weight training, 62
Cologne, 95, 98
Cooking, 135, 138
Cooldown, 10, 31, 54
Cooper, Kenneth, 3
Coping, 121–29
Crunches, 20
Cycling, 51, 54, 56–58

DeCinces, Doug, 124
Dehydration, 62
Domres, Marty, 72
Double-leg half-squat, 29
Double-leg lowering lift, 30
Dress code of Baltimore Orioles, 107, 109, 111

Ectomorph, 111–12
Elbow and wrist stretch
    hand down, 42
    hand up, 42
Elbow pull
    behind back, 41
    behind head, 38, 41
Endomorph, 111
Exercise program, 2–3, 7–8
Exercise(s)
    posture/body balance, 72–75
    stretching. See Stretch(ing)
    types of, 8–9
    warmup, 10–11

Fats, 81–82
Flanagan, Mike, 123
Flat back, 71

Food groups, 85–86
Foods, 85–89
Frisbee, 57
Fruit-and-vegetable group, 86

Gibson, Kirk, 61
Golf, 56, 58
Grain group, 86
Groin stretch, 13, 15
Grossman, Ted, 88
Gymnastics, 58

Hair care, 100–4
Hair style, 101–3
Hamstring stretch, 17
Handball, 58
Hardin, Jim, 125
Havlicek, John, 8–9
Heart disease
    cholesterol and, 82
    running and, 54
Heart rate
    maximum, 31
    resting, 12
    target, 30
Heel raise, 29
Heel cord stretch, 16
Hip flexor muscles, 71
Home, Jim Palmer's, 134
Houk, Ralph, 126
Hug
    reverse two-arm, 13, 15
    single arm, 43
    two-arm, 13, 15
Hurdler, 18, 19
    reverse, 18, 19

Isokinetic exercises, 9
Isometric exercises, 9
Isotonic exercises, 9

Jackson, Reggie, 109
Jockey underwear, 140
Jogging, 51–54, 58. See also Running
Judo, 58
Juggle arms, 26, 27
Junk food, 86

Karate, 58
Kayak, 58
Kneading, 45, 47
Kneeling, 74

Leg lifts
    back, bent knee, 23, 25
    back, straight knee, 23, 25
    side, 22, 25

Leg lowering, partial, 20, 21
Leonhard, Davey, 2
Letterman, David, 125–26
Lifestyle, 2–3
Lifting weights, 62, 74
Liquids, 83–84
Lonborg, Jim, 51
Lower back, postural problems and, 72
Lying position, 73

McGraw, Tug, 125–26
Martial arts, 58
Meat group, 86
Medical checkup, 54
Mesomorph, 111
Milk group, 86
Minerals, 85
Moisturizer, 94, 95
Muser, Tony, 109, 111

Nautilus equipment, 60, 61
Neck bends, 12
Niekro, Phil, 9
Nutrition, 79–89
    calories, 81
    caarbohydrates, 83
    fats, 81–82
    food groups, 85–86
    liquids, 83–84
    minerals, 85
    protein, 82–83
    vitamins, 84–85
    weight loss and, 87–89

Overhead stretch, 13, 14, 72
Overtraining, 62–63

Paddle arms, 22, 24
Palmer, Jamie, 135, 138
Palmer, Kelly, 135, 138
Palmerfit program, 7–8
Pants, 111–12, 116
Pappas, Arthur, 38, 61–62
Parallel leg stretch, 16
Partial leg lowering, 20, 31
Partial sit-ups, 20, 73
Pelvic force couple, 71
Pelvic tilt, 19, 20, 73
Pelvis, 70
    level of, 73
Permanent, 103
Pitching, 1–2, 139–41
    stress and, 121–29
Polyunsaturated fats, 82
Posture, 69–75
Professional athletes, stress and, 121–29
Protein, 82–83

Punch up arms, 22, 24
Pushing and pulling, 73–74
Push-ups, 26
    three-hand-position, 48

Quad stretch, 16

Racquetball, 56, 58
Resistance training, 60–63
Restaurants, eating in, 80
Resting Heart Rate, 12
Reverse arm circle, 26, 27
Reverse hug, 72
Reverse hurdler, 18, 19
Reverse leg lift, 23, 25
Reverse two-arm hug, 13, 15
Roberts, Robin, 123
Rollover, 22, 23
Rowing, 58
Rugby, 58
Runner's build, 54
Running, 51–54, 58
    attire for, 52
    in cold weather, 52, 54
    heart disease and, 54
    surfaces for, 52
    talk test for, 52
    technique of, 52

Saturated fats, 82
Sawing
    front to back, 44, 45
    side to side, 45
Scents, 95, 98
Scuba, 58
Shampoos, 100–1
Shaving, 95
Shirts, 116
Shoes, 112, 116
Shoulder-blade pinch, 72
    number 1, 49
    number 2, 49, 51
    number 3, 50, 51
Shoulder roll, 44, 45
Shoulders, round, 71–72
Side bends, 13, 14, 26, 28, 73
Side hip stretch, 43
Side leg lifts, 22, 25, 73
Single-leg half-squat, 29
Sitting posture, 73
Sit-ups
    full, 20, 21
    partial, 20, 73
    V, 29
Skating, 59
Skiing, 51, 58–59
Skin care, 93–95

Skin diving, 58
Soap, 94–95
Soccer, 57, 59
Socks, 116
Softball, 57, 59–60
Sports, 37–63. *See also individual sports*
  one-on-one, 56
  playing, 51–60
  team, 56–57
  warmup program for, 38–51
  on your own, 51–56
Sports jackets, 116
Spring training, 88
Sprinter, 13, 16
Squash, 58
Squatting, 74
Stanhouse, Don, 102
Stooping, 74
Strength training, 60–63
Stress, 121–29
Stretch(ing), 11–18
  Achilles' tendon, 16
  airplane, 13, 15
  ankle circle, 38, 40
  arm crossover, 45, 46
  back, 18, 19
  back arm reach, palms turned in, 38, 41
  back arm reach, palms turned out, 38, 41
  ball roll, 48
  circular arm swing, 42
  elbow and wrist, hand down, 42
  elbow and wrist, hand up, 42
  elbow pull, behind back, 41
  elbow pull, behind head, 38, 41
  groin, 13, 15
  guidelines for, 12
  hamstring, 17
  heel cord, 16
  hurdler, 18, 19
  kneading, 45, 47
  neck bends, 12
  overhead, 13, 14
  parallel leg, 16
  sawing front to back, 44, 45
  sawing side to side, 45
  shoulder-blade pinch number 1, 49
  shoulder-blade pinch number 2, 49, 51
  shoulder-blade pinch number 3, 50, 51
  shoulder roll, 44, 45
  side bends, 13, 14
  side hip, 43
  single arm hug, 43
  three-hand-position push-up, 48
  twister, 12–13
  two-arm hug and reverse two-arm hug, 13, 15
Suits, 112, 114

Sunscreens, 99–100
Suntan, 98–100
Sweaters, 116
Swimming, 51, 54, 60

Table tennis, 60
Talk test, 52
Tanning, 98–100
Tennis, 56, 60
Three-hand-position push-up, 48
Ties, 114
Trousers, 111–12, 114, 116
T-shirts, 116
Twister, 12–13
Two-arm hug, 13, 15

Vitamin A, 84
Vitamin C, 85
Vitamin D, 85
Vitamin E, 85
Vitamins, 84–85
Vitamins B-complex, 85
Vitamin supplements, 85
Volleyball, 57, 60
V sit-up, 29

Walking, 51–52, 60
Warmup Chart, 32
  sports, 39–40
Warmups, 10–11
  cardiovascular and muscular-skeletal
    components of, 11
  sports, 38–51
  stretching exercises for. *See* Stretch(ing)
Water, 83–84
Water skiing, 60
Weaver, Earl, 103, 109, 125–27
Weight loss, 87–89
Weight training, 60–63
Windmill arms, 26, 28
Windmill stretch, 15
Workout chart, 33
Workout cycle, 4-week, 53
Workouts, 10, 18–29
  aerobic exercise activity, 30
  arm cirlce, 16, 17
  back leg lift, bent knee, 23, 25
  back leg lift, straight knee, 23, 25
  back lift, 26
  barbell arms, 22, 24
  bent knee-up or partial leg lowering, 20, 21
  biceps raise, 29, 30
  bow and arrow, 22
  double-leg half-squat, 29
  double-leg lowering lift, 30
  full sit-ups, 20, 21

Workouts *(cont'd.)*
  heel raise, 29
  juggle arms, 26, 27
  paddle arms, 22, 24
  partial sit-ups or crunches, 20
  pelvic tilt, 19, 20
  punch up arms, 22, 24
  push-up, 26

Workouts *(cont'd.)*
  reverse arm circle, 26, 27
  reverse leg lift, 23, 25
  rollover, 22, 23
  side bends, 26, 28
  side leg lifts, 22, 25
  single-leg half-squat, 29
  windmill arms, 26, 28

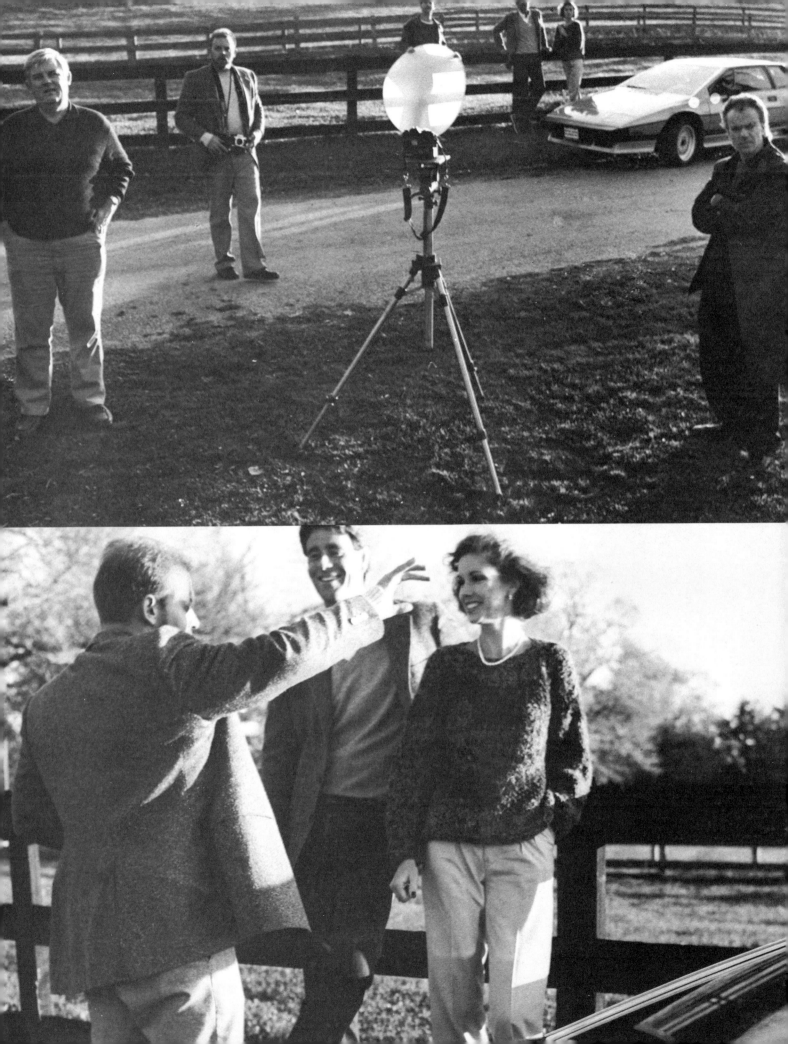

ACKNOWLEDGEMENTS

BEHIND THE SCENES

Chaos in repose? No, just a quintessential book-producing crew at work. The photographs on page 165 were snapped on location near Jim Palmer's Maryland home in late afternoon, November, 1984. The principals, who were waiting for the sun to position itself properly, are, in top photo, from lower left and clockwise: Jack Clary, writer/collaborator; Jon Naso, photographer; Bob Briody, assistant photographer; Jim Palmer, author; Diana Bergfeld, model; and Joe Montebello, art director, Harper & Row Publishers.

This cast was assembled to take photographs for the fashion segments of *Jim Palmer's Way to Fitness*, just one of a succession of tasks necessary to produce a book. Book producing is a growing phenomenon in book publishing. It is the creation, development and production of a book *outside* the normal operations of the contracting publishing house. This book was produced by Mountain Lion, Inc., which specializes in bringing health, fitness,

sports and professional books to market. A book producer brings together and relies on the special skills of many people. The following contributed to producing *Jim Palmer's Way to Fitness*, to whom we say, "Thanks."

- *Jack Clary,* writer, who collaborated with Jim to produce the text; and *Guy Kettelhack,* who assisted Jack.

- *Jon Naso,* photographer, who took both the brilliant color photographs for the jacket and black-and-white photographs for the text; and *Bob Briody,* who assisted Jon.

- *Nancy L. Siegel,* RPT, who designed the exercise programs, initially during Jim's active baseball career when he needed to recover from injury and most recently when we needed a consolidated regimen for this book; *Glenn Swengros,* Director of Program Development of the President's Council on Physical Fitness and Sports, and *Matt Brzycki,* Strength Coach of Rutgers University, who reviewed and refined the exercise programs; and *Eileen Berl Eisenberg,* M.S., R.D., who developed the nutritional guidelines.

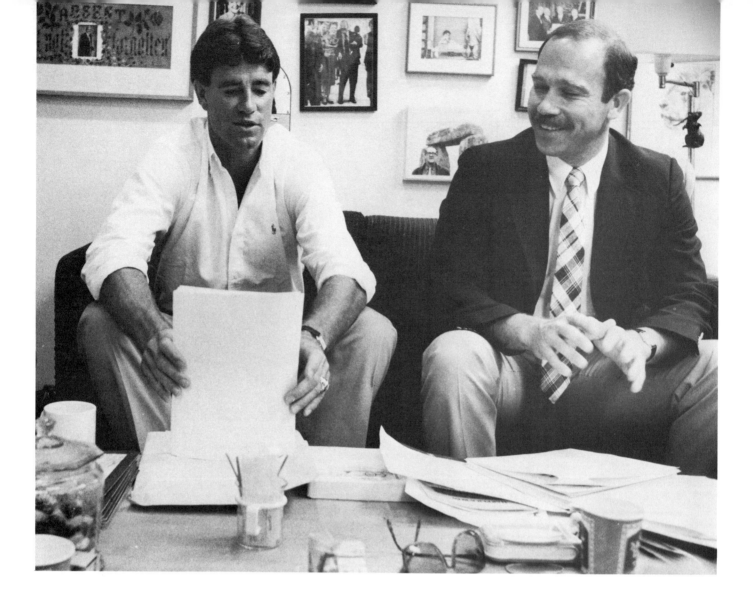

- *Larry Ashmead,* editor who shepherded the project for Harper & Row; *Margaret Wimberger,* editorial assistant who helped Larry; and *Joseph Montebello,* art director, who coordinated the photography, jacket and book design, and, on location, Jim's clothing for the camera.

- *Matt Merola,* Mattgo Enterprises; *Lynn Watner* and *Ron Shapiro,* Personal Management Associates—agents all, and *Jim Fox* and *Jon Gaynin*—attorneys who helped put together the principals.

- *Doris Tucker* of Mountain Lion Inc. and *Vivian G. Raskin,* The Office in Owings Mills, who, respectively, typed the manuscript and transcribed the many taped interviews; and *Bill Laznovsky,* Mountain Lion, Inc., who helped edit the photographs.

- Also: *Rik Davis,* Codalight Studio, N.Y. City; *Erica Feinberg,* Erica Feinberg Associates, N.Y. City; *Scott Propper,* President, The Motor Coach, Ltd., Baltimore, Md., *Yvette Blasco,* Lillian Lehman Co., E. Brunswick, N.J.; *Diane Bergfeld,* Central Casting, Baltimore; *Bill Herman,* Jockey International; *Bob Little,* Butler Aviation-Baltimore/Washington, Inc., *Paul Goucher,* Libco, Inc., Mountainside, N.J.

John J. Monteleone
Mountain Lion Inc.
Rocky Hill, N.J.
January, 1985

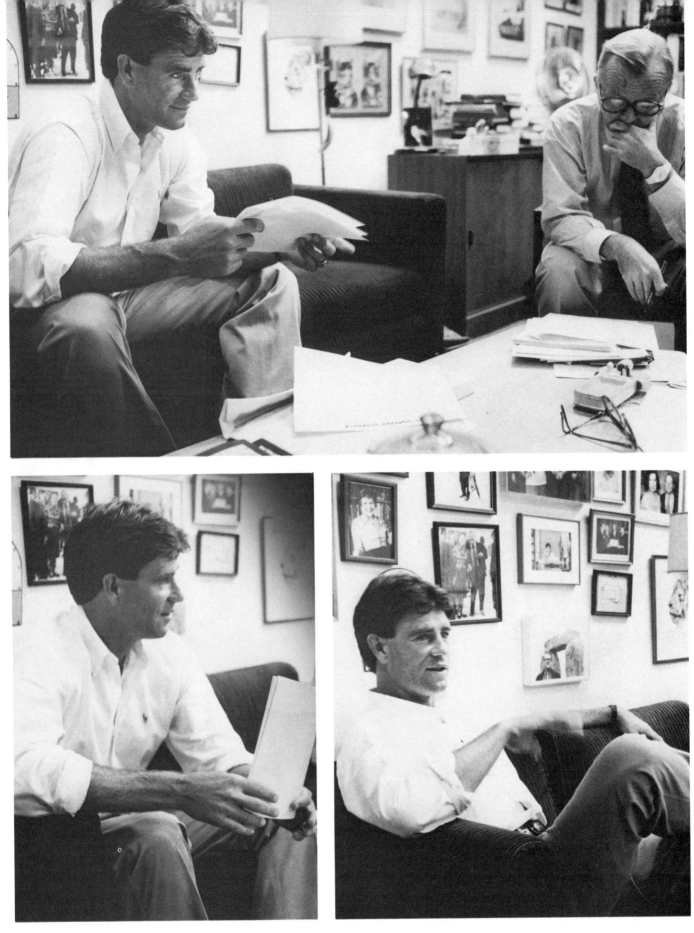

Jim Palmer: "He has the best 20-year-old body in baseball," Earl Weaver, former Baltimore manager once remarked about the then-more-than-30-year-old Palmer. "When rookies ask what to do in spring training, I say, 'Follow Palmer.' No one has ever kept up with him." Now retired from baseball, Palmer is still in constant motion. As a spokesman for Jockey International, sportscaster for ABC-TV and PBS, parent of two teenaged daughters, Jamie and Kelly, avid fitness practitioner and amateur athlete, Palmer seldom pauses to sit and relax in his comfortable suburban Baltimore home. In fact, now just entering his forties, he seems to be picking up momentum. But one will be able to intercept him one afternoon in August, 1989, his first year of eligibility for induction into the Baseball Hall of Fame, in Cooperstown, N.Y. when he stops by to join the other greats of the game.

Jack Clary: A freelance writer/author with more than a dozen books on sports to his credit, Clary's most recent collaboration is the bestselling *The Art of Quarterbacking* by Cincinnati Bengal Ken Anderson. His other works include *Careers in Sports, Pro Football's Great Moments, The Gamemakers* and coauthorship with Paul Brown of that famed coach's autobiography, *PB.*

Clary worked for seventeen years as a daily journalist and columnist for The Associated Press, New York *World Telegram & Sun* and Boston *Herald Traveler,* and is a regular contributor to *PRO!* magazine.

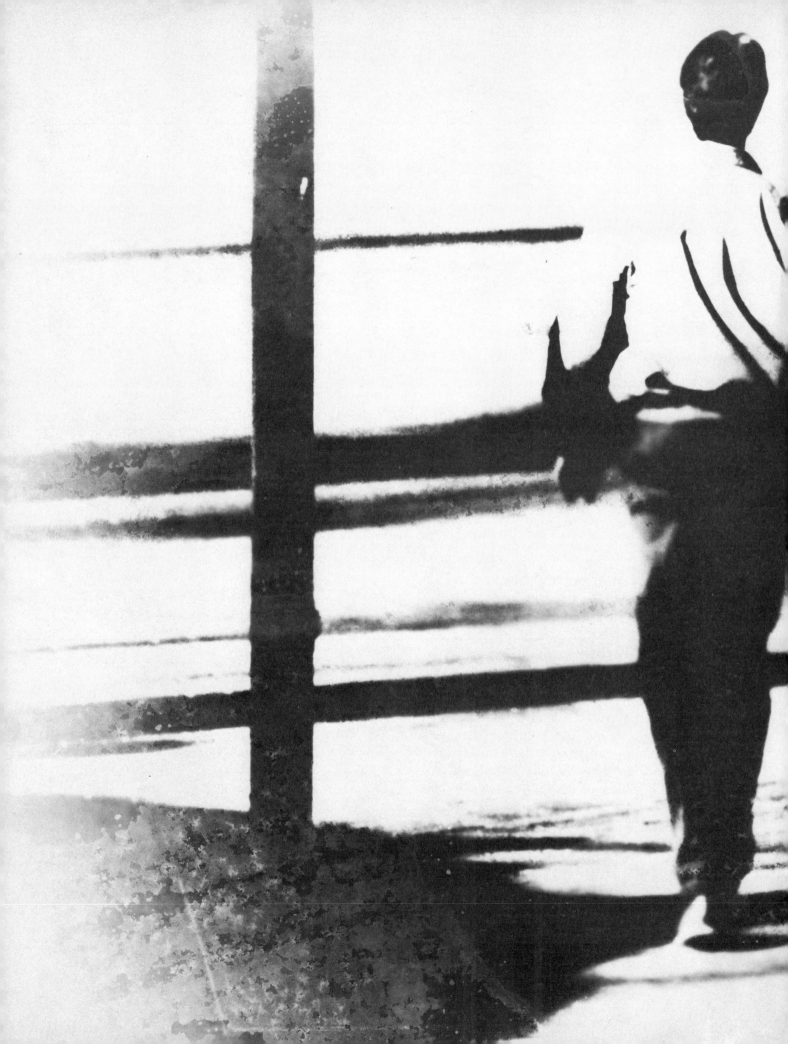